Comorbid Eating Disorders and Obsessive-Compulsive Disorder

Comorbid Eating Disorders and Obsessive-Compulsive Disorder

A Clinician's Guide to Challenges in Treatment

Jenna DiLossi
Center for Hope & Health, LLC, Pennsylvania

Melissa Harrison
Center for Hope & Health, LLC, Pennsylvania

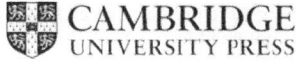

CAMBRIDGE
UNIVERSITY PRESS

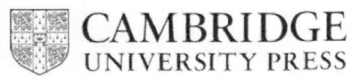

Shaftesbury Road, Cambridge CB2 8EA, United Kingdom

One Liberty Plaza, 20th Floor, New York, NY 10006, USA

477 Williamstown Road, Port Melbourne, VIC 3207, Australia

314–321, 3rd Floor, Plot 3, Splendor Forum, Jasola District Centre,
New Delhi – 110025, India

103 Penang Road, #05–06/07, Visioncrest Commercial, Singapore 238467

Cambridge University Press is part of Cambridge University Press & Assessment,
a department of the University of Cambridge.

We share the University's mission to contribute to society through the pursuit of
education, learning and research at the highest international levels of excellence.

www.cambridge.org
Information on this title: www.cambridge.org/9781009186872

DOI: 10.1017/9781009186865

First published 2024

A catalogue record for this publication is available from the British Library

Library of Congress Cataloging-in-Publication Data
Names: DiLossi, Jenna, author. | Harrison, Melissa (Counselor), author.
Title: Comorbid eating disorders and obsessive-compulsive disorder : a clinician's guide to challenges in treatment
/ Jenna DiLossi, Center for Hope & Health, LLC, Pennsylvania, Melissa Harrison, Center for Hope & Health, LLC,
Pennsylvania.
Description: Cambridge, United Kingdom ; New York, NY : Cambridge University Press, 2024. | Includes
bibliographical references and index.
Identifiers: LCCN 2023025916 (print) | LCCN 2023025917 (ebook) | ISBN 9781009186872 (hardback) | ISBN
9781009186872 (paperback) | ISBN 9781009186865 (ebook)
Subjects: LCSH: Compulsive eating. | Obsessive-compulsive disorder. | Eating disorders.
Classification: LCC RC552.C65 D55 2024 (print) | LCC RC552.C65 (ebook) | DDC 616.85/26–dc23/eng/20230622
LC record available at https://lccn.loc.gov/2023025916
LC ebook record available at https://lccn.loc.gov/2023025917

ISBN 978-1-009-18687-2 Paperback

Contents

Part I Overview of the Existing Literature

Part II Clinical Pitfalls and Treatment Failures

Part III Evidence-Informed Considerations for Assessment and Treatment

Part IV Special Topics and Future Considerations

Foreword

Obsessive compulsive disorder is a common condition that confers significant impairment and risk of considerable psychiatric morbidity and attenuated quality of life. Despite this, the field has been fairly impressive in that the available treatment options are very effective in both clinical trial and applied settings. More specifically, cognitive-behavioral therapy with exposure and response prevention (CBT) and pharmacotherapy with serotonin reuptake inhibitors have demonstrated significant benefit for adult and pediatric patients with OCD. Notable across the research literature is inclusion of individuals with OCD who have a wide range of comorbidities – with a couple notable exceptions.

People with comorbid eating disorders have been excluded in most prior OCD treatment trials and posed a clinical challenge for practicing clinicians treating individuals with OCD. Yet, disordered eating symptoms are quite common in people with OCD as well as the other way around. This presentation has historically been a sort of "kryptonite" for practicing clinicians, and the fields of OCD and eating disorders became split in a sense. Eating disorder clinicians would often struggle to effectively treat OCD with evidence-based psychotherapy and OCD clinicians would hesitate to enter into treatment with patients who had active eating disorders. A large part of this was the lack of guidance available with regards to how to treat this comorbid presentation. Another factor was that past eating disorder treatments were at times theoretically inconsistent with evidence-based intervention for OCD patients. As a result, a great many individuals were inadequately treated, compounding continued distress and suffering.

DiLossi and Harrison have made a notable contribution to the literature to effectively remedy this issue. "*Comorbid Eating Disorders and Obsessive-Compulsive Disorder: A Clinician's Guide to Challenges in Treatment*" synthesizes all that practicing clinicians need to know in order to effectively understand and treat comorbid eating disorders and OCD. The authors have truly thought of it all in this book. Chapters focus on recognizing eating disorder and OCD presentations, conceptualizing treatment from a cognitive-behavioral standpoint, engaging other healthcare professionals and family members, intervention implementation, and addressing pitfalls. The book thoughtfully starts off with a discussion of both clinical presentations, successfully capturing the intricacies of each condition as well as their comorbid presentation. Discussion of the nature of treatment, mechanisms of action, and clinical pitfalls are spot on target and impressive for their clarity – something that will be particularly helpful for clinicians who are new to either of these presentations. In fact, a major strength of the book is its practical nature in detailing the various aspects necessary for successful treatment. For example, text focuses on engaging other healthcare providers, and designing meal plans consistent with a CBT-based approach. Notable inclusions also involve how to do effective exposures as well as understanding what 'less' effective exposures may look like and various missteps that therapists can make in treating these conditions. DiLossi and Harrison convey their considerable expertise in guiding the reader to understand not only how to effectively treat this comorbid presentation but also how to identify problems and pitfalls, and effectively address them. Clinical vignettes bring the text to life and facilitate the reader in imagining how to implement clinical techniques.

The field of OCD and eating disorders have independently come a long way but – until now – a void has remained in how to treat comorbid eating disorder and OCD presentations. DiLossi and Harrison have effectively addressed this issue by providing a clearly written, expert handbook based on evidence-based principles of psychological intervention. This text will become a go to resource for practicing clinicians and should be on the bookshelf for clinicians working with people with eating disorders and/or OCD. There is no doubt that this text will serve as a vehicle for improving wellness of many people who are struggling with this co-occurring presentation.

Eric A. Storch

Baylor College of Medicine, Department of Psychiatry &
Behavioral Sciences, Houston, TX

Disclosure Statement

Eric Storch reports receiving research funding to his institution from the Ream Foundation, International OCD Foundation, and NIH. He is a consultant for Brainsway and Biohaven Pharmaceuticals. He owns stock less than $5000 in NView. He receives book royalties from Elsevier, Wiley, Oxford, American Psychological Association, Guildford, Springer, and Jessica Kingsley.

Preface

This book was born out of an amalgamation of challenges that we have seen in practice over the years. We both started off our training as eating disorder (ED) therapists and, throughout our years in practice, we noticed many gaps between what the research had been indicating and what we saw implemented in the field. Before we had training and experience providing evidence-based treatment to clients, we ourselves made many mistakes and engaged in the therapist drift (Waller, 2009). After seeking training for empirically driven treatments, we became passionate about the provision and dissemination of evidence-based care.

Once we began implementing evidence-based treatments for EDs (i.e., CBT-E, FBT) we were impressed by the results. Specifically, we saw the power and fulfillment of providing exposure-based techniques within these treatments. At the same time, we observed a significant overlap of EDs with anxiety disorders and traits of obsessive-compulsive disorder (OCD). In fact, there was a patient who was very successful in her treatment for anorexia nervosa (AN) where regular eating, weight exposures, challenging food myths, and shifting her values facilitated great progress. One problem, however, was that in creating dissonance between her strong value for animal rights and her fear of carbohydrates in her ED (leading her to eat a lot of protein and little carbohydrates), her value-driven treatment plan encouraged her to eat vegetarian in recovery. This quickly backfired when we began to realize that not only was it a value not to eat animals, but that she had morality-based OCD. Missing an OCD diagnosis and not understanding the nuances of the comorbidity was one of the catalysts to seek more formal anxiety and OCD training. A few years into our training, we truly began to see the high degree of overlap between EDs and OCD . . . and began to realize what we may have missed over the years in our patients. Not only did we notice the overlap, we also noticed that these individuals seemed to have poorer outcomes in ED treatments, and appeared to have struggles that persisted and/or worsened as a result of various interventions within ED treatment.

In looking at the existing research, we found that the phenomenological overlap and diagnostic comorbidity was well documented. In fact, it is estimated that up to 60% of patients with EDs will have a lifetime history of OCD (Godart et al., 2002, 2003; Halmi et al., 2005; Kaye et al., 2004). Research has also noted how co-occurring OCD may complicate treatment or yield less favorable outcomes (Byrne et al., 2017; Lock & Le Grange, 2019; Vall & Wade, 2015; Wentz et al., 2009). OCD and EDs create complex treatment challenges and, despite the frequency of comorbidity, very little has been written or researched to dictate treatment (Simpson et al., 2013). In other words, to date there are little to no guidelines indicating what clinicians ought to do with this presentation in clinical practice to improve outcomes.

This conundrum became particularly relevant to our practice as our referral base for co-occurring cases grew due to us having specialized training in both disorders. We were tasked with extrapolating from the existing literature on these disorders, our clinical hunches, and observations from mistakes made in the past to best treat these individuals. We are so grateful to our patients, who have trusted our training and clinical judgment, and to our colleagues, who have provided consultation over the years.

The purpose of this book is threefold. First, we want to provide an overview of what the research has demonstrated thus far about how to conceptualize and treat stand-alone and comorbid EDs and OCD. Second, we want to highlight the gaps in the literature regarding best practices for treating this comorbid presentation and offer evidence-informed insights into the clinical pitfalls and treatment failures that clinicians commonly encounter when treating patients with both disorders. Third, we want to offer clinicians evidence-informed considerations for assessment and treatment to better account for the comorbid presentation and likely improve overall treatment outcomes. In doing so, we will also provide some additional considerations on special topics to inform future research and practice.

This book is intended to serve as a supplemental resource for clinicians to use in treatment alongside existing empirically supported treatment manuals when the comorbidity is present. It also aims to provide a platform to inform future research, as it is our hope that some of the topics and suggestions mentioned here could help to inform development of a systematic treatment protocol. Furthermore, we want to make clear that this book is not intended to be viewed as a validated systematic protocol (as its suggestions have not been empirically tested), but rather as a supplemental guide for clinicians in practice.

Thank you very much for your interest in our book and for your dedication to helping your patients with this co-occurring presentation. It is our sincerest hope that this book will be of use to you in your practice.

Acknowledgments

We would like to extend our heartfelt gratitude to all those who have supported and encouraged us in the writing of this book. Thank you to our partners, Tristan and Kyle, our parents, and our friends – your unwavering support and encouragement has meant everything to us. We are also so grateful to our dedicated staff, including but not limited to, Liia, Meghan, Paulina, Alyssa, and Christina, who have been instrumental in the writing process. Thank you to our esteemed colleagues who have trained us and supported our goals and growth in different ways, including Suzanne Straebler, MaryAnn Layden, Rebecka Peebles, Eric Storch, Nick Farrell, Carolyn Becker, David Yusko, Steven Tsao, and Sandy Capaldi, along with those who have been gracious in their dissemination efforts, especially those at Oxford University. Thank you to the editors at Cambridge University Press, including Sarah Marsh and Kim Ingram, who made the book a reality. This book would not have been possible without the support and encouragement of so many people, and we are truly grateful to each and every one of you.

Last but not least, a special thanks to the patients who have shared their stories, worked hard in treatment, and proven with bravery and grit that recovery is possible. Your resilience and strength have inspired us, and we are honored to have had the opportunity to be a part of your journeys.

Abbreviations

ADHD	attention deficit hyperactivity disorder
AN	anorexia nervosa
APA	American Psychiatric Association
ARFID	avoidant/restrictive food intake disorder
AS	anxiety sensitivity
BDD	body dysmorphic disorder
BED	binge-eating disorder
BMI	body mass index
BN	bulimia nervosa
BPD	borderline personality disorder
CBT	cognitive-behavioral therapy
CPS	child protective services
CT	cognitive therapy
DBT	dialectical behavioral therapy
DT	distress tolerance
EA	experiential avoidance
ED	eating disorder
EDNOS	ED not otherwise specified
EPT	emotional processing theory
ER	emotional regulation
ERP	exposure and response prevention
FBT	family-based treatment
FPT	focal psychodynamic therapy
GAD	generalized anxiety disorder
ICAT	integrative cognitive affective therapy
ILT	inhibitory learning theory
IU	intolerance of uncertainty
MDD	major depressive disorder
MI	motivational interviewing
NU	negative urgency
OCD	obsessive-compulsive disorder
OCRD	obsessive-compulsive-related disorders
ON	orthorexia nervosa
OSFED	other specified feeding or eating disorder
PIOS	Penn Inventory of Scrupulosity
PTSD	post traumatic stress disorder
RCT	randomized controlled trials
RP	response prevention
SSCM	specialist supportive clinical management
SSRI	selective serotonin reuptake inhibitor
TAF	thought–action fusion
TSF	thought–shape fusion
YBOCS	Yale–Brown Obsessive-Compulsive Scale checklist

This section aims to broadly review the main topics of the book, and the corresponding existing literature. In addition to an overview of EDs and OCD (and their empirically supported treatments), this section is intended to highlight the common overlap and similarities found in the disorders, in addition to the prevalence of comorbidity. It is also intended to inform the purpose of the book by highlighting gaps in the literature pertaining to treatment recommendations. There is a particular focus on synthesizing the key features that these treatments have in common. We believe that it is particularly important to highlight these key features as pillars to guide effective treatment, given that there is not a validated systematic protocol to follow at the current time.

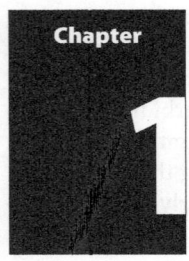

Understanding Eating Disorders

Eating disorders (EDs) are serious biological, psychological, and culturally based disorders that are widespread in many parts of the world. They are relatively common psychiatric disorders and, although rates vary, some estimate the lifetime prevalence of EDs to be 8.4% for women and 2.2% for men worldwide (Galmiche et al., 2019). EDs are life threatening and cause psychological impairment as well as substantial life dysfunction (American Psychiatric Association [APA], 2013). Medical comorbidities (e.g., cardiac arrhythmias, osteoporosis, gastroenterology issues, infertility) and high suicide rates are associated with the disorder, leading to mortality rates up to five times higher than the general population (Yao et al., 2016).

EDs are treatable. Full recovery is possible, especially with early intervention (Mitchell et al., 1993; Treasure & Russell, 2011). However, many patients do not receive the care they need to recover (Keski-Rahkonen & Mustelin, 2016). EDs are associated with high levels of shame and stigma, partly because they are trivialized as vanity issues, which prevents individuals from seeking treatment (Becker et al., 2020). Additionally, specialist ED clinicians are not up to date on the best practices. In the United States, there is a dearth of clinicians trained in evidence-based treatment, which hinders patients from receiving the interventions needed for recovery (Cooper & Kelland, 2015; Waller et al., 2012). There is still more to be done in understanding EDs and with their respective treatments, especially considering there are still a number of patients in evidence-based treatment who don't show significant progress (Dalle Grave et al., 2013; Legenbauer & Meule, 2015). Understanding why people are not getting better is critical to amending treatments and improving recovery rates.

In an effort to provide a comprehensive understanding of this overlapping presentation, this chapter provides a brief overview of the EDs typically seen to co-occur with OCD. The following sections outline the criteria for EDs, along with their key features, maintenance variables, and a brief overview on the treatments that are most indicated. Chapter 2 will provide a detailed understanding of the leading treatments for EDs.

Classification of EDs

The *Diagnostic and Statistical Manual of Mental Disorders – Fifth Edition* (DSM-5) has reorganized the way EDs are classified. The new categorization, named Feeding and Eating Disorders, expanded diagnostic criteria for most EDs. Binge-eating disorder (BED) was officially added and the residual diagnostic category previously named ED not otherwise specified (EDNOS) was expanded and renamed other specified feeding or ED (OSFED). The EDs discussed in this book include anorexia nervosa (AN), bulimia nervosa (BN), BED, avoidant/restrictive food intake disorder (ARFID), and OSFED.

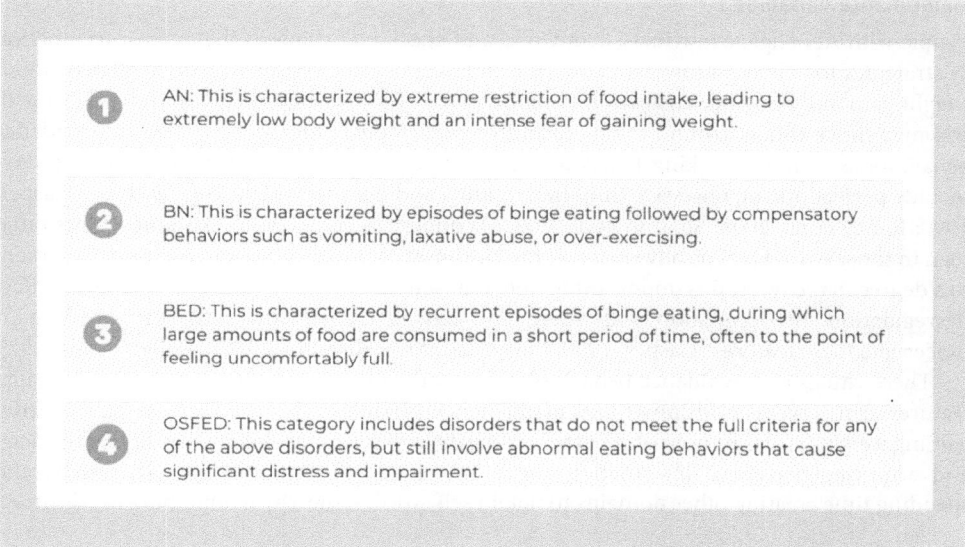

① AN: This is characterized by extreme restriction of food intake, leading to extremely low body weight and an intense fear of gaining weight.

② BN: This is characterized by episodes of binge eating followed by compensatory behaviors such as vomiting, laxative abuse, or over-exercising.

③ BED: This is characterized by recurrent episodes of binge eating, during which large amounts of food are consumed in a short period of time, often to the point of feeling uncomfortably full.

④ OSFED: This category includes disorders that do not meet the full criteria for any of the above disorders, but still involve abnormal eating behaviors that cause significant distress and impairment.

Figure 1.1 Classification of EDs

AN Presentation

AN is a psychiatric disorder characterized by food restriction leading to a significantly low body weight or lack of appropriate weight milestones. AN is associated with an intense fear of weight gain, a marked disturbance in body image illustrated by significant body dissatisfaction and/or body dysmorphia, and poor insight regarding the seriousness of the current low body weight and/or the behaviors impeding weight gain. Two subtypes are recognized: the restricting type and the binge-eating/purging type (APA, 2013).

Key Features

Individuals with this disorder reach an extremely low weight by restricting the amount of food consumed, and, at times, by engaging in excessive exercise. Extreme restriction is achieved in three major ways: eating as little food as possible through methods such as counting calories, delaying eating for as long as possible (i.e., missing meals, fasting), and cutting certain foods or food groups out of their diets (e.g., desserts, fats) (Fairburn, 2013). People with AN may also misuse laxatives and/or diuretics, engage in self-induced vomiting, or exercise to manage weight and reduce anxiety about eating and weight gain (Fairburn, 2013). There are also a number of personality or temperament features often observed in people with AN: perfectionism (Halmi et al., 2000; Shafran et al., 2002), high harm avoidance, high obsessionality (Le Grange et al., 2012), and overall high trait anxiety are often present (Pollice et al., 1997). These traits may serve as clues to the risk factors, shared neurobiological or genetic links with other disorders (e.g., behavioral phenotype of OCD), and explanations for some of the difficulties in responding to treatment (Strober, 2004).

Maintenance Variables

People with AN engage in rituals, avoidance, and checking behaviors that appear to function as strategies to achieve a lower weight, prevent weight gain, and/or to reduce anxiety about weight gain and body dissatisfaction (Gianini et al., 2015; Steinglass, 2011). Individuals with AN may move things around the plate and/or meticulously measure their food. Avoidance behaviors as well as checking behaviors are common. Personality traits in those with AN include perfectionism, obsessive thinking, rigidity, and use of avoidant coping styles (Casper, 1990; Raney et al., 2008; Shafran et al., 2002; Wonderlich et al., 2005). Although traits often seen in those with AN typically exist prior to the onset of the disorder and can remain present to a degree in recovery, it is important to note that starvation effects (e.g., obsessionality, affect dysregulation, preoccupation with food) and having the AN diagnosis can produce or exacerbate these features (Casper, 1990; Kaye et al., 2004; Keys et al., 1950; Pollice et al., 1997).

These rituals and avoidance behaviors, along with effects from starvation and personality features, can serve as both onset and maintenance variables. They prevent the patient from gaining weight (and thus nourishment), building distress tolerance skills, violating expectancies and acquiring corrective information about how food affects the body and anxiety, and spending time creating other domains to obtain self-worth – thereby maintaining the disorder.

AN Treatment

Empirically supported treatments for adults with AN are limited. There is a lack of evidence pointing to one psychological treatment emerging as superior for adults with AN (Byrne et al., 2017; Dalle Grave et al., 2016; Watson & Bulik, 2013), and there is no current evidence for pharmacology providing an alternative (Cassioli et al., 2020). The psychological treatments that have some evidence for change include the Maudsley model of AN treatment for adults (MANTRA), cognitive-behavioral therapy enhanced for EDs (CBT-E), specialist supportive clinical management (SSCM) (Byrne et al., 2017; Dalle Grave et al., 2016; Zeeck et al., 2018), and focal psychodynamic therapy (FPT) (Zeeck et al., 2018). None of these treatments have provided impressive outcomes thus far. In 2017, Byrne et al. compared MANTRA, SSCM, and CBT-E. All three treatments showed an equivalent reduction in psychopathology with no significant differences with regard to BMI change. However, CBT-E was more effective in helping patients achieve a physically healthy weight. Further, a study by Fairburn et al. (2013) on CBT-E for adult AN demonstrated improvements in weight and ED pathology. This study provides strong, promising support for CBT-E and its transdiagnostic application.

Treatment outcomes for adolescents with AN are more robust, resulting in clear treatment recommendations, including family-based treatment (FBT) as the gold standard and CBT-E adapted for adolescents as a reasonable alternative (Dalle Grave et al., 2013; Lock & Le Grange, 2019).

BN Presentation

BN is characterized by binge eating followed by a compensatory behavior to prevent weight gain and to avoid any physical and/or psychological consequences of the binge (e.g., bloating, guilt). Binge eating is defined as consuming an unusually large amount of food within a short period of time (within two hours), accompanied by a perceived loss of control to stop eating or inability to limit the food intake. Compensatory behaviors can include

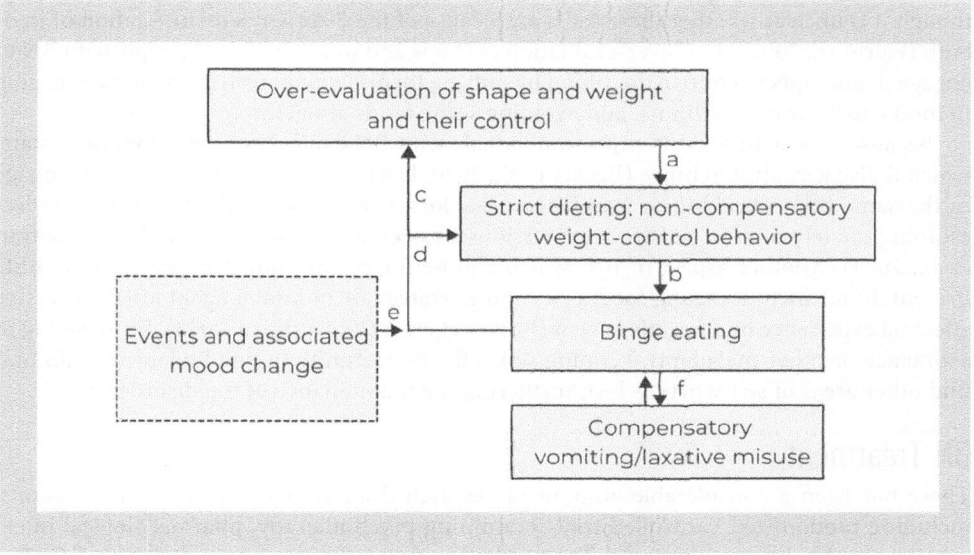

Figure 1.2 Binge Cycle

purging via self-induced vomiting or inappropriate laxative use, as well as nonpurging compensatory behaviors such as excessive exercise, fasting, diuretics, or any other medications to prevent weight gain. Additionally, self-evaluation is unduly influenced by body shape, weight, and their control (APA, 2013).

Key Features

Individuals with BN engage in dietary restraint but may slip and break a "rule" or eat something regretful with family or peers due to social pressure. Subsequently, they may experience intense regret and negative self-talk, which then can lead to maladaptive behavior, including bingeing. People with BN often experience all-or-nothing/black-and-white thinking about food: for example, "I already screwed up, so I might as well just keep eating." Overeating is often perceived as a failed attempt to diet, which is associated with feeling like a failure. The person might then continue to eat or binge to escape the negative feelings associated with the perceived failure.

Individuals with BN have a higher incidence of other impulsive maladaptive behaviors, including alcohol abuse, shoplifting, and self-harm behaviors, as well as comorbid disorders such as depression, personality disorders, and substance use disorders (Crow et al., 2014; Godart et al., 2002; Hatsukami et al., 1986; Vervaet et al., 2004). Impulsivity, novelty seeking behavior (Atiye et al., 2015), emotional dysregulation, and struggle with distress tolerance (Anestis et al., 2007; Lavender et al., 2015) are also common.

Maintenance Variables

The best-understood model for conceptualizing the key features and maintenance factors for BN has been described by Fairburn (2008). Similar to AN, those with BN spend a lot of time and energy trying to lose weight, prevent weight gain, and attain an ideal body. People with BN have an overemphasis on weight, shape, and the control thereof on their self-worth, though it is unclear whether these traits are a cause of the disorder, a manifestation of it, or both (Fairburn, 2008). This over-evaluation of shape and weight will lead people with BN to engage in attempts to control their food by putting themselves on restrictive diets, engaging in food rituals or calorie limits, and avoiding some foods altogether.

Because of weight loss attempts, individuals with BN can be in a semistarvation state, which is also a catalyst to binge (Becker et al., 2020; Fairburn, 2013). They also often engage in the same body checking or avoidance behaviors as those with AN, which may reflect escaping anxiety and/or be direct expressions of overvaluing weight and shape (Shafran et al., 2004). Another aspect of BN, which will be further examined in the section "BED Presentation," includes using food as a coping strategy or numbing agent after a negative affectual experience or a negative event (Becker et al., 2020; Fairburn, 2013). By engaging in avoidance or other maladaptive coping skills, the opportunity to build adaptive skills and find other areas of self-worth is lost, furthering the maintenance of the disorder.

BN Treatment

There has been a considerable amount of research done on treatment of BN in adults, including randomized controlled trials examining psychotherapy, pharmacological interventions, and their combinations. The results have consistently demonstrated that CBT is superior to other forms of psychotherapy for adults (Poulson et al., 2014; Shapiro et al., 2007). Interpersonal psychotherapy (IPT) is considered a leading, empirically supported alternative to CBT according to the National Institute for Health and Clinical Excellence (NICE, 2020), and there has been some promising research on the effects of dialectical behavioral therapy (DBT) on BN (Chen et al., 2008; Safer et al., 2010).

There is evidence suggesting that the combination of CBT paired with an antidepressant medication (typically a selective serotonin reuptake inhibitor [SSRI]) can lead to optimal outcomes for some adults with BN (Agras et al., 1992; Walsh et al., 1997). However, CBT alone has been shown to produce the largest treatment effect (Flament et al., 2012; Hagan & Walsh, 2021). While a thorough review of pharmacological treatments is not the focus of this book, high doses of the SSRI fluoxetine is approved by the FDA to treat BN in adults specifically (Goldstein et al., 1995). For adolescents, research outcomes provide similar suggestions to the treatment of adolescent AN, where FBT is the leading recommendation and CBT-E adapted for adolescents is a reasonable alternative (Dalle Grave et al., 2013; Lock & Le Grange, 2019).

BED Presentation

Individuals with BED engage in the same binge-eating behavior as those with BN, but with an absence of compensatory behaviors. As mentioned, a binge involves consuming excessive amounts of food in a short period of time (e.g., within two hours), with a sense of loss of control of eating during the episode. Binge-eating episodes are associated with three or more of the following: eating more rapidly than normal, eating until uncomfortably full, eating large amounts when not physically hungry, eating alone with a sense of embarrassment, feeling disgusted with self, depressed, or very guilty afterward. The diagnosis of BED does not require there to be an overemphasis on weight, shape, their control, and/or body image concerns (APA, 2013).

Key Features

BED impacts many people; some estimates concluding that it has the highest prevalence of all EDs (Erskine & Whiteford, 2018), but it is often clandestine as the majority of people do not seek help (Coffino et al., 2019b). Keski-Rahkonen (2021) describes several large studies where binge eating was found in people with a history of abuse, neglect, and violence. Perceived or real excess weight, childhood weight-related teasing, body dissatisfaction, and persistent dieting are shared risk factors for binge eating across all socioeconomic groups (West et al., 2019). Although there is an absence of the overvaluation of shape, weight, their control, and/or body image difficulties as a diagnostic criterion, it is still a commonly occurring cognition and has been found to be correlated with higher levels of ED psychopathology (Grilo et al. 2008; Hrabosky et al., 2007). Further, Coffino (2019a) found that this overvaluation of weight and shape was associated with greater BED-related functional impairment.

Maintenance Variables

Similar to those with BN, people with BED may overeat and perceive this way of eating as a failure, leading to all-or-nothing thinking as well as a shame and guilt mindset. This emotional state can then fuel subsequent binge eating. Bingeing can result from not consuming enough food throughout the day. Lack of adequate nutrition can result from dieting, but also from stress-induced appetite loss, poor planning, or issues with appetite-regulating hormones (Fairburn, 2013). Ultimately, bingeing may be a result of dietary suppression or it may serve as a pure coping strategy for different mood states or negative life events. These behaviors and coping styles quickly become cyclical and self-maintaining. Those with higher weights who have internalized the erroneous (and fatphobic) belief that people have higher weights because of an internal trait or personal deficit (e.g., lack of self-discipline) will be particularly susceptible to this cycle of dieting or feeling shame around food choices and amount of consumption (Durso et al., 2012).

BED Treatment

Both CBT and IPT have demonstrated strong empirical support for BED (Wilson et al., 2007). For pharmacology, the only drug currently approved for BED is lisdexamfetamine dimesylate. For a more comprehensive review on pharmacology, see Brownley et al. (2007) and Reas and Grilo (2015).

ARFID Presentation

ARFID is characterized by an eating or feeding disturbance leading to a condition associated with one or more consequences, including significant weight loss, poor growth, nutritional deficiency, psychosocial dysfunction, or the need for supplemental nutrition. Individuals with ARFID do not avoid or restrict food based on a body image disturbance or undue emphasis of weight, shape, or their control. The eating issue is not associated with cultural or religious practices, cannot be attributed to a medical condition, and does not occur during the course of AN or BN (APA, 2013).

Key Features

ARFID can present in a number of ways; however, there are typically three primary reasons why most patients report avoiding food: (a) fear of aversive consequences of eating;

(b) long-standing reduced appetite, quick to feel full, and/or a lack of interest in food; or (c) sensory discomfort. A patient may fear that they will vomit, choke, and/or feel physical discomfort in certain areas of the body when eating. Additionally, patients may have an aversive reaction to certain food textures, temperatures, colors, or smells, or have a preoccupation with how food is served (e.g., foods that are touching or how food is cut) and how it is prepared (e.g., vegetables need to be cooked lightly to still retain crunchy sensation) (Nicely et al., 2014; Thomas et al., 2018).

This feeding or eating disturbance is associated with extreme selective eating, appetite disruption, sensory sensitivities, or anxiety. Individuals diagnosed with ARFID often have experienced pickiness or feeding issues beginning in childhood or infancy, have comorbidities that also include sensory sensitivity traits (autism spectrum disorder [ASD], attention deficit hyperactivity disorder [ADHD], intellectual disabilities), and/or have a co-occurring anxiety disorder where there is a long history of engaging in safety and escape behaviors to manage anxiety (Nicely et al., 2014; Spettigue & Norris, 2019). Patients, and/or their parents, may use language such as "eats like a bird" or "does not really like food" to describe the patient's relationship with food.

Maintenance Variables

Patients of all presentations behave with rigidity and avoidance, as well as using rituals and/or safety/escape behaviors. Often, parents or partners will accommodate the avoidance by making a separate meal to the rest of the family or allowing exceptions in school to meet the patient's expressed "needs." Similar to other EDs, the symptoms of anxiety, appetite suppression, and hypersensitivity to sensory elements can be exacerbated by the starving or semistarvation state, thus maintaining or worsening the disorder (Nicely et al., 2014). Additionally, avoidance (directly by the patient or indirectly through accommodation from a loved one) will maintain the patient's low self-efficacy in their ability to tolerate the discomfort triggered by the food. Avoidance and safety behaviors will also maintain the fears around adverse consequences like vomiting and choking. As a result, the patient has less opportunity for inhibitory learning and to develop tolerance to uncertainty and distress (Thomas & Eddy, 2018).

ARFID Treatment

There are no well-established, empirically supported treatments for ARFID (Lock, 2015). Prospective research and conclusions drawn from studies have suggested that FBT, parent-support models, CBT, exposure-based interventions, and adjunctive pharmacology may attain the best results (Dalle Grave & Sapuppo, 2020; Thomas et al., 2020). A feasible and acceptable CBT manual for medically stable outpatient ARFID patients (CBT-AR) has been developed. A feasibility study done on CBT-AR for adults demonstrated a large and significant increase in BMI, and at posttreatment 47% of patients no longer met the criteria for ARFID. The authors note that randomized controlled trials are needed to confirm findings, but results suggest promising outcomes (Thomas et al., 2021).

OSFED Presentation

When someone is experiencing eating disturbances that cause clinical distress or life impairment in important areas of functioning but the behaviors do not meet full criteria for an ED listed in the DSM-5, they will receive an OSFED diagnosis. The categories proposed include atypical AN (AN without significant low weight), purging disorder (recurrent purging to influence shape or weight with the absence of binge episodes), and night eating syndrome (binge eating occurring exclusively at night, usually associated with sleep issues). The subthreshold disorders include clinically significant disordered eating that does not meet full criteria for AN, BN, or BED (e.g., BN or BED with frequency of binge episodes less than once per week) (APA, 2013).

In the DSM-5 there is also a category named Unspecified Feeding or ED (UFED). This diagnosis is provided when the symptoms are clinically impairing or distressing but there is not sufficient information to make a definite diagnosis, or when the clinician chooses not to identify the reasons why the criteria for a disorder are unmet. Other disordered eating problems exist. They do not have formal recognition but can cause significant impairment and psychological distress. One of these unclassified disorders relevant to the topic of this book is orthorexia nervosa (ON). ON involves an extreme preoccupation with healthy eating.

Originally described by Bratman (1997), ON is characterized by inflexibility with food, ritualized eating patterns, food avoidance, and food elimination driven by a concern around food being unhealthy or impure. There is an absence of an official diagnosis and lack of uniformity and methodology issues in assessment; however, there seems to be enough evidence to support ON as a separate disorder (Dunn & Bratman, 2016). Dunn and Bratman (2016) have proposed diagnostic criteria that include an obsessive focus on "healthy" eating, evidenced by compulsive behavior or mental preoccupation around restrictive dietary practices to optimize health, a violation of self-imposed dietary rules causing exaggerated fear of disease, a sense of personal impurity, and or physical sensations accompanied by anxiety and shame. Dietary restriction can become more rigid and intense over time, typically leading to weight loss despite an absence of this desire. The aforementioned traits cause clinical impairment in at least one meaningful area.

Key Features

This disorder clinically presents as an overlap of AN and OCD features (Missbach et al., 2017). Similar to AN, patients typically have low insight into how their behaviors are maladaptive or a denial of the consequences of their rigid eating. Further, they will eat with similar rituals, attempt to control all food preparation (e.g., avoid eating at restaurants, bring prepped meals to social events), practice reading labels to look for specific ingredients, use food scales, count macronutrients, eliminate certain foods or food groups, and display distress if they cannot engage in these behaviors. Eventually, people experience medical and psychological consequences such as low body weight, malnutrition, and relationship or occupational stress from the prioritization of or preoccupation with "health" over other areas of functioning.

Maintenance Variables

Individuals with ON have self-worth that is often tied to successfully complying with their food rules, and they may feel superior to others based on their diet. Similar to OCD, patients will have intrusive obsessions about health that cause anxiety and distress largely based on irrational or improbable fears (although reinforced by culture and media). They demonstrate low tolerance for eating in any way that may jeopardize their "health" and engage in compulsions including rituals, mental reviewing (e.g., thinking about all the "clean eating" choices made over a period of time), reassurance seeking (e.g., asking loved ones if they believe the food they're consuming is healthy), and avoidance to either prevent becoming less "healthy" or to reduce their anxiety about health. This naturally functions to reinforce their rigid beliefs about health and food. This process becomes exhausting and time consuming, and creates dysfunction in many areas of the person's life.

ON Treatment

There is scant literature providing little direction for any empirically supported treatments for ON. However, considering the overlapping features of AN and OCD seen in ON, treatment options may be ascertained from the empirically supported treatments of these similar disorders. This notion points to some version of exposure-based CBT, with some family assistance for adolescents. Further literature and scholarship are needed to provide more direction for treatment.

In Summary

EDs are a group of mental health conditions characterized by abnormal eating habits and distorted attitudes toward food and body weight. EDs can affect people of all ages, genders, and backgrounds, but they are more common in females and typically begin in adolescence or young adulthood. They often involve a preoccupation with weight, body shape, and diet, and can lead to severe and dangerous weight loss, as well as having serious physical and psychological consequences (e.g., malnutrition, organ damage, death). Risk factors for EDs include a history of dieting, low self-esteem, perfectionism, and a history of trauma or abuse. EDs often co-occur with other mental health conditions, such as anxiety, OCD, depression, and substance abuse. EDs are treatable, and study outcomes have indicated CBT, FBT, IPT, and (in some cases) medication as the leading treatments for these disorders. Co-occurring presentations, especially OCD, can engender complexities, including those that affect and impair treatment.

Review of Eating Disorder Treatment

There are a number of options for treating EDs. Broadly, there are options relating to the treatment setting, including inpatient stays, residential treatment, partial hospitals, and outpatient care. There are also different therapeutic orientations (e.g., psychodynamic, interpersonal psychotherapy), as well as questions around the use of ancillary treatments (e.g., nutritional counseling, movement therapy). The current literature indicates that unless the patient is medically compromised, at risk of suicide, has not experienced improvement on an outpatient level, or there is a significant hindrance or danger in the home (i.e., abuse, unsafe living environment), the least restrictive environment is ideal and often produces the best outcomes when utilizing evidenced-based treatment models (Meads et al., 2001; Zeeck et al., 2009). Thus, we will be summarizing outpatient treatments with the most information and their respective research. We will provide more detailed descriptions of the treatments that are more behavioral in nature and therefore most relevant to this comorbidity. This knowledge will prepare you for a comprehensive understanding of the shared etiology between EDs and OCD and provide suggestions for more inclusive treatment.

FBT

Theory

FBT is an empirically supported manualized treatment for adolescent EDs originating from the work of Christopher Dare and Ivan Eisler at the Maudsley Hospital in London, and later advanced and manualized by Daniel Le Grange and James Lock. FBT holds an agnostic outlook on the illness with no assumptions regarding the origin of the disorder. It integrates techniques derived from different schools of psychotherapy, including systemic, Milan, strategic, narrative, and structural family therapy. Targeting ED symptoms and weight gain early in treatment may help patients by quickly reducing starvation effects. Many behaviors and cognitions associated with AN could be attributed to the result of starvation, which has been documented famously in the classic Minnesota Starvation Studies (Keys, 1950) where increased obsessionality and psychopathology resulted from reduced caloric intake. Although weight gain may be a primary mechanism of action in FBT, Lock and Nicholls argue that weight gain cannot be the only mechanism of action considering the high relapse rate post-inpatient treatment where weight gain is often achieved. FBT encourages the family to externalize the illness, operating from the perspective that the child is not capable of making healthy decisions related to food and the ED thoughts are impeding normal adolescent development (Dalle Grave et al., 2019; Lock & Nicholls, 2020). FBT empowers the family to become a resource and a primary agent of change in the recovery of the adolescent (Le Grange et al., 2015). As the cognitions and behaviors associated with the ED remit, more time is spent on typical adolescent anxieties, including fears around weight gain and eventually things like dating, applying to college, individuation from parents, and so forth.

Treatment Description

The treatment is typically delivered in three distinct phases that include approximately 10–20 sessions over a period of 6–12 months. For those with AN, the first stage centers on weight gain, wherein the primary caregivers take control of the child's food (e.g., cooking all meals, serving and monitoring all meals, choosing meal plans). The therapist takes time to increase the caregiver's self-efficacy in their role by providing information, observing a family meal, and continuing to coach the family to hold a noncritical, compassionate stance while remaining firm during mealtime. For adolescents with BN, there is a more collaborative approach to behavioral change between the patient and parent. This greater collaboration can occur because BN patients have more awareness of symptomatology and less cognitive impairment compared to AN patients (Loeb & Le Grange, 2009). When a minimal weight is achieved or bulimic symptoms have reduced, stage two begins. The second stage focuses on helping the parents transition food control back to the child. There is an increased focus on eating while socializing and eating in more typical environments than the home (e.g., restaurants, school cafeterias). Other issues that could not be resolved because of previous weight gain goals (e.g., social anxieties, family conflict) can now begin to be reviewed. Finally, stage three focuses on more age-appropriate problems and preparing for termination (Lock & Le Grange, 2013).

Empirical Support

FBT is the first-line treatment option for adolescents with AN and BN and has shown early promise in treating children with ARFID (Lock et al., 2019). FBT has been tested in a number of randomized controlled trials and has demonstrated efficacious results, especially in populations where the patients are younger and have a shorter duration of illness. For those with AN, results estimate a 75% treatment response for improvement in weight and eating-related psychopathology (Lock & Le Grange, 2019). For adolescent BN, 40% of participants achieved remission (defined as abstinence from bingeing and purging for four consecutive weeks prior to assessment) in the two studies that have utilized manualized FBT-BN (Le Grange et al., 2007, 2015; Lock & Le Grange, 2019).

Despite FBT being the leading empirically supported intervention for adolescent EDs, it is not without limitations. For example, parents who are overly critical of their children in treatment have poorer outcomes (Le Grange et al., 1992). Similarly, data also suggests that FBT appears less effective and efficient when there are obsessive-compulsive features present (Lock & Le Grange, 2019). Overall, the less than ideal response rates combined with an approach that is sometimes not feasible or suitable for families leaves room for alternative approaches.

Cognitive-Behavioral Therapies for EDs (CBT-ED)

Current forms of evidence-based CBT for EDs include CBT-E, CBT-guided self-help (CBT-gsh), 10-session cognitive-behavioral therapy (CBT-T), and CBT for ARFID (CBT-AR). The relevant evidence-based forms of CBT-ED (Fairburn, 2008; Waller et al., 2018b) are structured, manualized, and based in behavioral change, particularly around eating and body (e.g., reducing dietary restriction, body checking).

CBT-E

Theory

CBT-E is an empirically supported treatment for BN and BED in adults that has shown promising results for adolescent AN (Dalle Grave et al., 2013). Christopher G. Fairburn developed a CBT treatment protocol for BN (CBT-BN) in the late 1970s. Later, with the help of colleagues Zafra Cooper and Roz Shafran, he observed that many patients with other EDs shared similar core psychopathology, and he developed an enhanced transdiagnostic treatment that could be applied to all EDs (Cooper & Fairburn, 2011). CBT-E focuses on the core psychopathology of overvaluation of body weight, shape, and their control, and targets the maintenance variables of the illness. Additional variables such as core low self-esteem, clinical perfectionism, and interpersonal difficulties are also thought to maintain the pathology for some people (Fairburn, 2008). Consistent with most CBT, the process of remitting the ED must be collaborative, with patients showing motivation and a willingness to stay committed to treatment. The patient and therapist collaboratively use behavioral interventions (e.g., collaborative weighing, self-monitoring) and strategically planned homework to achieve change.

Treatment Description

CBT-E in its most used form (i.e., the focused form: CBT-Ef) consists of four stages that are typically delivered in 20 sessions over the course of 5 months or 40 sessions for 9 months for underweight or restrictive disorders. Early success is a significant predictor of positive treatment outcome (Fairburn, 2008); thus, appointments are twice-weekly in stage one. Patients receive psychoeducation and motivational interviewing to ensure willingness to stay engaged in treatment. Stage one also prioritizes eating stabilization via collaborative in-session weighing, self-monitoring, and establishment of regulated eating. For AN patients, weight gain is a target, while for BED and BN patients the formulation includes events and mood changes as a trigger to binge eating, as well as a compensatory behavior for BN. Stage two is a transitional stage used to identify individual difficulties and barriers to success, and to plan which variables should be targeted in stage three. Stage three is the core body of treatment and seeks to address the primary maintaining variables of the individual's ED (i.e., overevaluation of body image, events/mood changes, dietary restraint). Stage four focuses on sustaining progress and minimizing risk of relapse to achieve long-term change (Fairburn, 2008). CBT in its lesser-utilized form (the broad form, CBT-Eb) extends to roughly 10 added sessions, or longer sessions (80 minutes versus 50 minutes), and addresses the additional variables thought to maintain the eating pathology (i.e., core low self-esteem, clinical perfectionism, and interpersonal distress).

Adapted for Adolescents

CBT-E for adolescents is largely identical to the treatment for adults but includes modifications for age and development (Cooper & Stewart, 2008) and a more thorough motivational process (Dalle Grave et al., 2019). Parents are brought in for psychoeducation and then invited for check-ins, eventually leading to some joint sessions. Parents can be utilized to help problem-solve barriers, increase adherence to behavioral interventions, and keep the home environment conducive to recovery (Dalle Grave et al., 2019).

Empirical Support

Initial data from a cohort study found that approximately 60% of treatment completers achieved a full response with CBT-E (Dalle Grave et al., 2019). A recent nonrandomized effectiveness trial comparing FBT and CBT-E in adolescents suggested that both treatments are solidified as viable options (Le Grange et al., 2020).

CBT-Guided Self-Help (CBT-gsh)

CBT-gsh is a manualized, lower-intensity treatment for adults with mild to moderate BN/ BED. It is based on the principles of CBT-E and involves a facilitator guiding the person through self-help program materials in order to change unhelpful thinking patterns and behaviors related to their disordered eating or ED. CBT-gsh is recommended as an afford-able and cost-effective evidence-based psychological intervention for adults with BN and BED (NICE, 2020). CBT-gsh typically consists of 10–20 sessions that can be delivered face-to-face or online, and takes 25–50 minutes per session. The frequency and intensity of the sessions may vary depending on the individual's treatment plan and progress (Fairburn et al., 2009, 2015; Linardon et al., 2017; Wilson & Zandberg, 2012).

Empirical Support

CBT-gsh therapies may be as effective as other active therapies for BED (Wilson & Zandberg, 2012) and a useful treatment for BN (Linardon et al., 2017; Wilson et al., 2007). In a meta-analysis, CBT-gsh was consistently more effective than inactive comparisons (i.e., waitlist) (Linardon et al., 2017; Sysko & Walsh, 2008). Wilson et al. (2010) found that CBT-gsh demonstrated equal effects on binge-eating pathology and behavior compared to IPT and behavioral weight loss treatment effects. More research is needed, but given the efficacy and easy dissemination, paired with the reduced cost, CBT-gsh treatments should be considered as an option for patients.

CBT-T

CBT-T is a 10-session manualized outpatient treatment for patients with EDs who have a body mass index (BMI) above 17.5. It incorporates elements of CBT for EDs, such as in-session weighing, exposure therapy, nutrition education, cognitive restructuring, body image work, and relapse prevention. It is intended to be delivered by novice therapists, such as provisional psychologists, under specialist supervision.

Empirical Support

CBT-T has promising preliminary research. A study of 106 patients in the United Kingdom found that CBT-T resulted in statistically and clinically significant reductions in both behavioral and cognitive measures of ED symptoms, as well as improvements in secondary outcomes such as depression and anxiety. It demonstrated a substantial reduction in eating and related pathology similar to existing treatments that are twice as long (Fairburn et al., 2009; Waller et al., 2014, 2018a). A subsequent case series also replicated these findings (Pellizzer et al., 2019; Waller et al., 2018a).

IPT

IPT for EDs is a structured and time-limited treatment for adults with BN and BED, adapted by Christopher Fairburn from IPT for depression. It is based on the idea that how a person relates to others can affect their emotional and mental health, and therefore their ED symptoms. IPT helps people to develop an understanding of the relationship between their interpersonal problems and their ED symptoms, and then works to help them identify and resolve key relationship-based factors that are maintaining their ED symptoms. This is done through interventions such as learning to handle conflict, loss, transition, and relational difficulties. The goal of IPT is to help people establish a sense of themselves as part of a supportive and accepting social context that provides an alternative to their ED for seeking positive self-esteem and emotional well-being. IPT is typically delivered in 12–20 sessions over a period of 4–6 months. It is intended for adults over the age of 18 with BN or BED (contraindicated for AN).

Empirical Support

IPT and CBT are both equally effective for binge-related behaviors and cognitions. IPT has empirical support for the treatment of adult BN and is considered the leading alternative to CBT-E (Agras et al., 2000; Fairburn et al., 2015; Hagan & Walsh, 2021; Karam et al., 2019). There are a few studies comparing CBT and IPT directly, and both treatments have reliably shown to significantly reduce binge-eating symptoms and associated pathology, as well as demonstrating lasting recovery in follow-ups (Karam et al., 2019; Wilfley et al., 1993, 2002; Wilson et al., 2010). Wilson et al. (2010) found that CBT-gsh and IPT emerged as superior when looking at sustaining effects during follow-up appointments (Wilson et al., 2010; Wilson & Zandberg, 2012).

CBT for ARFID (CBT-AR)

CBT-AR is an emerging treatment option for individuals aged 10 and older with all presentations of ARFID who are medically stable and not reliant on tube feeding. Developed at Massachusetts General Hospital, CBT-AR is a structured, time-limited out-patient intervention that can be delivered in an individual or family-supported format, lasting between 20 and 30 sessions depending on the degree of nutritional compromise. CBT-AR focuses on volume before variety to support nutritional rehabilitation (i.e., weight gain) and uses structured in-session exposure to address maintaining mechanisms relevant to the patient (Thomas et al., 2018).

Empirical Support

While efficacy data is not yet available, preliminary results are promising in terms of weight gain, resolution of nutrition deficiencies, and modest expansion of dietary variety in case studies (Thomas et al., 2017).

In Summary

There are several treatment options for EDs that have been shown to be effective, including FBT for adolescents, CBT-ED for adults with BN and ED, and CBT-E for adults with AN and as an alternative to FBT. These treatments vary in their approach, but have similar outcomes. Understanding the common factors between these treatments and their potential barriers and mediators can help in the development of new treatments for comorbidity.

Understanding Obsessive-Compulsive Disorder

OCD, formerly characterized as an anxiety disorder (APA, 2013), impacts roughly 1–2% of the general population (Clark, 2020). This disorder is characterized by a pattern of obsessions and/or compulsions. The obsessions and compulsions are time consuming and intrusive, so much so that they affect daily functioning and cause considerable distress. Obsessions and compulsions are associated with many emotions, including anxiety (that may lead to panic attacks), shame, guilt, distress, profound sadness, emptiness, and uneasiness. OCD is also known to be present with many comorbid disorders, most commonly major depression disorder (MDD), EDs, anxiety disorders, and posttraumatic stress disorder (PTSD). Studies also show a strong association between suicidal thoughts and OCD (Balci & Sevincok, 2010).

The frequency and intensity of symptoms vary among patients with OCD. Some have mild to moderate symptoms (i.e., three–four hours per day), while others have severe obsessions and compulsions (i.e., eight or more hours throughout the day). Further, patients vary in the degree to which they believe that their obsessions and compulsions are unreasonable. The degree of insight varies; however, most patients realize that their obsessions and compulsions are dysfunctional or unreasonable. Similarly, some patients' symptoms present as ego-syntonic (e.g., obsessions about morality), while others have obsessions that are ego-dystonic (e.g., obsessions about pedophilia). Presentations with low insight and ego-syntonic obsessions tend to correlate with poorer treatment outcomes (Clark, 2020).

Classification of OCD

Since the 1980s, and until recently, behavioral and cognitive-behavioral theory, research, and treatment have conceptualized OCD as an anxiety disorder. Although minor changes occurred by way of diagnostic criteria, the DSM-5 (APA, 2013) reclassified OCD in its own category, accompanied by body dysmorphic disorder (BDD), hoarding disorder, trichotillomania, and excoriation disorder. This reclassification met with controversy, as research both supports and refutes the notion that OCD is qualitatively distinct from anxiety disorders.

The underlying mechanisms of action in both the psychological treatment (i.e., exposure and response prevention [ERP]) and the pharmacological treatment (i.e., SSRIs) work to reduce OCD symptoms by targeting the same variables that maintain anxiety. Much like the importance of understanding the relationship between worry and safety behaviors in anxiety disorders, successful management of OCD symptoms requires a thorough understanding of the relationship between obsessions and compulsions.

Key Features

Obsessions

By nature, obsessions are intrusive, unpleasant, and upsetting, and typically present in the form of images, thoughts, ideas, or impulses. Most people have occasional intrusive thoughts but ordinarily chalk them up to "weird" or "random" thoughts and ultimately dismiss them as meaningless (Rachman & DeSilva, 1978). In other individuals, these thoughts are assumed to have great significance, thereby causing greater anxiety and developing into an obsession. In addition to intrusiveness, other core features of how individuals respond to obsessions are unacceptability, resistance, and perceived uncontrollability (Clark, 2020). OCD clinicians often explain such responses as an effect of having a "sticky brain," whereby those with OCD get "stuck" on one of such thought by giving it meaning. In other words, individuals with OCD experience psychological distress and anxiety as a result of interpreting the presence of a thought, image, or impulse as something noteworthy about their character or the future.

Compulsions

Compulsions are characterized by repetitive or excessive behaviors/rituals or mental acts that are done in an attempt to reduce the obsessions and alleviate the associated fear or disgust. Compulsions also aim to prevent some type of feared outcome from occurring (e.g., death) or achieve a standard that is "just right." OCD convinces patients that performing such acts is the only way to either prevent a catastrophic outcome and/or alleviate the distress brought on by the obsessions. Often to the frustration of OCD patients, they feel compelled to perform such rituals even when they have insight into their irrationality. Regardless of their level of insight, compulsions often do effectively alleviate distress in that moment, thereby becoming reinforcing. Many patients fall into a cyclical path of obsession > heightened distress > compulsion > relief > obsession > heightened distress > compulsion > relief, and so on. Notable in this cycle is that, unbeknownst to the patient, compulsions provide only short-term relief and typically exacerbate obsessions over time. As obsessions intensify, compulsions often expand and become more time consuming.

Avoidance

Many patients will also engage in behavioral avoidance. They may avoid people, situations, and other stimuli that trigger obsessions and compulsions For example, patients who have harm-based obsessions, such as hitting people, may avoid going to social gatherings or even leaving their home. Avoidance functions as an attempt to preemptively escape the distress associated with obsessions and the series of compulsions that *must* occur after exposure to the stimuli that triggers obsessional content. Many patients with OCD are unaware of the true degree of their avoidance, often failing to catch all the subtle ways avoidance manifests in their day-to-day lives. While intended to improve functioning by sidestepping distress, avoidance prevents the patient from living their life. Ultimately, it prevents practicing distress tolerance, uncertainty tolerance, and violating expectations about fears. Life interference and functional impairment are then further exacerbated in presentations with many co-occurring subtypes.

Subtypes

OCD is widely accepted as a heterogeneous disorder that has varied presentations and many subtypes that may or may not change over time. As per the Yale–Brown Obsessive-Compulsive Scale checklist (YBOCS; Goodman et al., 1989), symptoms present in one or more of the following domains: harm (aggression), contamination/cleaning/washing, sexual, symmetry/exactness/ordering/arranging, religiosity/scrupulosity/morality, hoarding/collecting, somatic, checking, repeating, counting, and miscellaneous. While it is not uncommon for many individuals with OCD to experience distress related to at least two of these domains simultaneously, others may experience one of these domains as the "primary" source of distress at a given time.

Contamination/Cleaning

Fear related to contamination is one of the best-known presentations of OCD in popular culture; this presentation occurs in up to 50% of OCD patients (Hasler et al., 2005; Jalal et al., 2020; Mathes et al., 2020; Rasmussen & Eisen, 1992). The contamination subtype can best be understood as an excessive concern with dirt or germs or other stimuli that are typically associated with these contaminants. Typical stimuli include one or more of the following: (a) bodily secretions (i.e., urine, feces, saliva, or blood), (b) dirt, (c) variables linked to illness (i.e., germs, viruses, bacteria), (d) sticky substances or residues (i.e., glues or sticky food items), (e) possibly harmful household items (i.e., cleaning agents, chemicals, or detergents), (f) environmental chemicals (i.e., asbestos, mold, radiation, pesticides, or toxic waste), and (g) particular animals or insects (Clark, 2020). Humans' preference to avoid such stimuli and/or the inherent aversion to them is arguably evolutionary in nature (Curtis et al., 2011).

Distress can be due to both the implication of said contaminant (e.g., a bed bug getting in a suitcase in a hotel room and then infesting the person's home) or simply disgust (Williams et al., 2013). An individual may not have a fear related to a contaminant other than that it is "gross," "disgusting," or "dirty." Researchers (e.g., Williams et al., 2013) argue that contamination obsessions related to disgust may be more difficult to treat compared to obsessions related to contamination with a feared outcome. In contrast to fear-based obsessions, disgust-based obsessions require one to tolerate an unpleasant emotional state for an unknown period (Clark, 2020), and often decrease in treatment via exposure due to habituation and inhibitory learning (Craske et al., 2014).

Patients manage this obsession in one of two ways: excessive cleaning/washing of themselves and/or their possessions, or avoidance of people, places, and things wherein the probability of encountering germs/dirt is high (e.g., amusement park rides, hotel rooms, touching doorknobs, airplanes/subway trains, etc.). Furthermore, many will utilize a combination of compulsions and avoidance to quiet their obsessions. Between prolonged avoidance and the generalization of fears, the list of feared stimuli can grow with time. Not only do individuals with this subtype have difficulty tolerating the uncertainty of their feared outcome occurring, they also considerably overestimate the likelihood of the outcome happening (Clark, 2020).

Symmetry/Exactness

A fixation on exactness, symmetry, ordering, and arranging is a subtype of OCD that can also be understood as an excessive need for things to be "just right." It is one of the most commonly reported symptom clusters in OCD samples and nonclinical samples alike;

however, it is the least likely to be associated with depression, life interference, and help-seeking (Fullana et al., 2010). Pietrefesa and Coles (2008) suggest that this subtype is based on sociocultural norms, but when symptoms become extreme, the connection to cultural norms is lost. Uniquely, rather than being motivated by fear or anxiety, this subtype is motivated by a core feature of incompleteness (Bragdon & Coles, 2017; Clark, 2020; Cougle et al., 2013; Rasmussen & Eisen, 1992; Schulze et al., 2018). Summerfeldt (2004) described incompleteness as a worrisome feeling or state of discontent that one's actions, surroundings, or current state is "just not right." It is associated with sensory-affective disturbances, physical discomfort, and checking compulsions (Fornés-Romero & Belloch, 2017; Summerfeldt et al., 2015). Additionally, this subtype tends to present as more dispositional and trait-like, related to perfectionism and linked to aesthetic preferences for balance. Such findings have particularly noteworthy implications for treatment due to the underemphasized role of cognitions, appraisals, and beliefs in the construct of incompleteness (Clark, 2020).

Body-Focused Obsessions

Per the YBOCS (Goodman et al., 1989), somatic obsessionality is a broader category that more commonly refers to intrusive thoughts and compulsions related to one's physical sensations and bodily functions. The content within obsessions could range from fears that one has an existing illness that has not been identified yet to a fixation on one's blinking or breathing. Such obsessions are commonly related to the body's aesthetic or physical health. With the exception of body dysmorphia, it seems as though this niche presentation of body-focused obsessions has not been examined much in the current literature.

Repugnant Obsessions

OCD symptoms that center around religion, God, morality, ethics, and integrity fall under a broader category of repugnant obsessions. This category also includes obsessionality related to aggression; harm to self or others; sexual orientation; and forbidden, disgusting, or harm-based sexual thoughts or images (Clark, 2020). Guilt and shame are also commonly associated with repugnant obsessions; this is especially applicable in the case of repugnant obsessions that occur within the domains of religious scrupulosity and morality (Berle & Starcevic, 2005; Hale & Clark, 2013).

Religious Scrupulosity

Scrupulosity, as defined by Abramowitz et al. (2008), refers to religious beliefs and practices that turn into disturbing, stressful preoccupations, and compulsive rituals that are motivated by fear of a possible punishment. Individuals who are afflicted with religious scrupulosity are often terrified of having committed some type of "sin" via their thoughts, words, actions, or by failing to "please God." There are two common themes within the presentation of scrupulosity: (1) impurity and uncleanliness that leads to cleaning compulsions, and (2) concern over liturgy that often leads to repeating of rituals or prayers, confessing, or other means of reassurance (Greenberg et al., 2001).

Overall, research points to highly religious people as having greater fears about God, concern about committing a sin, increased guilt, and a higher presence of beliefs that involve control over thoughts, responsibility, and perceived threat (Abramowitz et al., 2002; Hale & Clark, 2013; Inozu et al., 2014; Sica et al., 2002). Thus, it is not surprising that religious obsessions are more common in religious people. However, religious obsessions can also present in agnostic and nonreligious individuals (Tek & Ulug, 2001). Perhaps the most relevant key to exacerbating the distress and impairment brought on by scrupulosity is one's intolerance for uncertainty (Abramowitz & Jacoby, 2014). The very nature of faith sets these individuals up for a never-ending cycle of doubt > fear > compulsion in that certainty related to sin, one's standing in God's eyes, one's fate after death, etc., is impossible to attain. Treatment aims to break this cycle by mitigating the fear-based association with religion so that individuals can embrace a faith-based approach to religion that aligns with their values.

Morality

The notion that morality is somewhat tied to the onset and maintenance of OCD has been widely supported (Doron et al., 2007, 2012; Reuven et al., 2014). This notion is particularly relevant in cases of repugnant obsessions, wherein patients cling to the uncertainty of "what I could be at my core" or "what I could do at some point in the future." The fear often involves some type of moral violation, leaving heightened doubt about one's true character and capabilities. Likewise, Clark (2020) argues that individuals with OCD are hypersensitive to perceived threats to their moral values. Compulsions serve to overcompensate for the "immorality" or "evilness" that may exist within one's true self. This manifests in real time as a pattern of constantly going out of one's way to serve others to prove that they are "a good person" to either oneself or others despite the absence of genuine altruism.

Consistent with research on religious scrupulosity, Doron and colleagues (2007, 2012) identified that these obsessions are associated with low moral self-perception. It is also not uncommon for obsessions of morality and religious scrupulosity to co-occur due to their shared theme of guilt (Berle & Starcevic, 2005; Doron et al., 2012). It should be noted that religious scrupulosity and morality obsessionality are not one and the same. Individuals without religious scrupulosity may still present with obsessions related to morality, ethical decision-making, and personal integrity. Often, the competing shame and guilt, as well as glorification and pride, involved in this subtype sometimes prevent the patient from seeking treatment.

Maintenance of OCD

OCD is no exception to the widely accepted notion that illnesses and injuries worsen over time when left untreated. Avoidance not only makes feared stimuli and situations feel scarier and more aversive over time, it also often impairs day-to-day functioning and, in severe cases, can lead to increased isolation. In the case of OCD, isolation prevents one from obtaining feedback from the world regarding the validity and utility of their beliefs and behaviors (i.e., corrective and inhibitory learning). Thus, it creates a perfect environment for symptom maintenance, poorer insight, and lower motivation to seek treatment. One's whole world can progressively be overtaken by the cycle of obsessions, compulsions, and avoidance when left untreated, resulting in impairment across multiple domains of functioning. Researchers have identified certain psychological correlates of OCD that are thought to maintain its symptoms.

Intolerance of Uncertainty

Intolerance of uncertainty (IU) was originally identified as a related variable in the pathogenesis of generalized anxiety disorder (Dugas et al., 1998, 2001). Gentes and Ruscio (2011) explain IU as a construct that presents across disorders, wherein a person experiences a negative mood state and a repetitive negative thought that revolves around some type of undesired outcome. Regarding OCD, IU involves a set of beliefs related to the need for attaining certainty, an inability to cope with unpredictable change, and difficulty with new situations (Obsessive Compulsive Cognitions Working Group, 1997 in Clark 2020). This construct is dimensional in nature and is believed to be a primary maintenance variable in OCD. The Intolerance of Uncertainty Scale consists of two dormant factors: a "desire for predictability" dimension and an "uncertainty paralysis" dimension. The former asserts that predictability is preferable and uncertainty is an unpleasant experience, whereas the latter implies that one is unable to function in situations of uncertainty (Birrell et al., 2011).

IU often manifests in checking and repeating compulsions, in addition to the overall time spent in the obsessive-compulsive cycle (Rachman, 2002; Tolin et al., 2003, 2009). It is important to note that checking compulsions can also present as mental acts wherein one repeatedly engages in mental reviewing. Bottesi and colleagues (2017) found that checking and repeating often continue until a sense of certainty or the "just right" feeling is achieved. Many patients with OCD hold unreasonable, unrelenting beliefs related to perfectionism; this will be further elaborated upon in Chapter 3.

Whether we realize it or not, the average person is forced to tolerate uncertainty about many domains of their life, some trivial and some important. Tolerating typos in emails, potential car accidents, chances of active shooters . . . the list of life's uncertainties is endless. Most of us tolerate these uncertainties without much notice on a daily basis. Those with OCD and a "stickier brain" often fixate on one or more of these uncertainties at various points in their life. What OCD chooses to fixate on is typically related to a person's values, identity, or morals (Veale, 2002).

Distress Tolerance (DT)

Distress tolerance, understood as a person's ability to manage both actual and perceived emotional stress, is often a struggle for those with OCD (Laposa et al., 2015). Despite the YBOCS capturing DT as part of OCD's presence, there has been little empirical examination of the direct associations between DT and OCD symptomatology. The existing empirical evidence that is available in support of its relationship with eating will be provided in Chapter 10.

As it relates to OCD, DT has been shown to predict the frequency of obsessions and the degree of increases in anxiety upon encountering obsessive-based stimulus (Cougle et al., 2011, 2013). While Laposa et al. (2015) identified a correlation between DT and OCD maintenance, they also noted that it was not a predictor of OCD symptom severity when anxiety sensitivity and IU were considered. Despite mixed findings, one thing we can assume about OCD and DT is that one's continued pattern of immediately complying with compulsive urges without resistance prevents the person from experiencing distress in the short-term. It is plausible to assume that this pattern only strengthens further obsessionality and weakens the "muscle" to tolerate distress in other domains of life as well. In fact, Jacoby and Abramowitz (2016) assert that improved DT is one of ERP's most valuable underlying mechanisms. It enables people to learn that their OCD concerns are inevitable parts of life that are nonthreatening overall.

Empirically Supported Treatments

Until the mid-1960s, OCD was thought to be resistant to both traditional psychodynamic psychotherapy and psychotropic medications. Similarly, early behavior therapies, such as systematic desensitization and aversion therapy, proved to be marginally successful at best. A breakthrough came in 1966 when Victor Meyer pioneered the technique of exposure and ritual prevention (used interchangeably and later referred to as exposure and response prevention [ERP]). Broadly, when researchers reference "CBT for OCD," it typically encompasses components from two of the most-studied psychological treatments for OCD: ERP and cognitive therapy (CT). Although researchers and practitioners continue to theorize about the ways in which OCD treatment could be enhanced with alternative psychotherapies (e.g., acceptance and commitment therapy) and psychotropic medication (e.g., add-on antipsychotics), the following review will include only treatments with notable empirical support.

Medication Management: SSRI

As this book is intended to help clinicians better navigate the psychological treatments relevant to comorbid OCD and EDs, an in-depth review of the neurobiology of OCD and mechanisms of action in SSRI treatment is beyond its scope. Therefore, the literature review provided here will briefly summarize the most notable findings on SSRIs pertaining to OCD symptoms and outcomes.

Empirical Support

SSRIs have been identified as quite useful in OCD treatment, according to several studies (e.g., Fineberg et al., 2013; Skapinakis et al., 2016) that have examined their efficacy in lessening the severity of OCD symptoms in addition to the depressive symptoms that often coexist. Their efficacy has been examined alone and in augmented CBT. When compared to placebo, SSRIs alone show a significant improvement in symptoms within the first two weeks. They are also associated with significantly lower relapse rates when taken long term (i.e., 24–52 weeks). Dosing is particularly important in terms of SSRI efficacy and OCD outcomes. Better outcomes tend to be associated with higher doses of SSRIs, although some SSRIs (e.g., escitalopram) could aid in relapse prevention. Furthermore, it is recommended that the highest effective dose be maintained for at least one year (Fineberg et al., 2013; Skapinakis et al., 2016).

Although such findings support the notion that SSRIs alone could be a suitable treatment for OCD, outcomes indicate that SSRIs alone are inferior when compared to CBT alone (Foa et al., 2005). SSRIs have also been deemed inferior to CBT as regards long-term effects. Studies have shown that 45–89% of patients who experienced improvements in OCD symptoms with SSRIs also experienced a return of symptoms after treatment was discontinued (Pato et al., 1988; Simpson et al., 2004). In recent years an expansive body of research (e.g., Krzyszkowiak et al., 2019) has shown that a combined approach of CBT and a high-dose SSRI yields the most robust positive outcomes. Lastly, all SSRIs (i.e., citalopram, fluoxetine, fluvoxamine, paroxetine, and sertraline) have been confirmed as efficacious without significant differences.

ERP

Theory

The theory of classical conditioning underlies the core interventions of ERP. Said theory asserts that neutral stimuli, including mental events or thoughts, can operate like a conditioned stimulus in that they can begin to elicit fear, anxiety, or distress when they are repeatedly paired with a naturally unpleasant stimulus (i.e., unconditioned stimulus). This reaction to the conditioned stimulus facilitates escape behaviors in the form of compulsions and avoidance because they reduce distress and anxiety. Despite short-term relief, these behaviors only strengthen the intensity of obsessions, which typically results in patients finding themselves in a self-defeating cycle of increasing intensities and frequencies over time. This cycle also strengthens faulty cognitions about the probability of danger and harm, the impact of said harm, one's ability to cope with distress, and the mechanisms that reduce anxiety. Behaviorists have highlighted several additional elements of learning (e.g., inhibitory learning, habituation, etc.) to explain the positive change seen in ERP. Such elements will be further explained in Chapter 6.

Treatment Description

In accordance with traditional CBTs contemporary, manualized ERP includes session agendas, a collaborative therapeutic relationship, psychoeducation, self-monitoring, homework outside of session, and relapse prevention. It is unique in that it also incorporates specific interventions (e.g., the fear hierarchy) that target the core mechanisms that maintain OCD. The original model of ERP developed by Meyer (1966) consisted of only in vivo exposure and ritual prevention. It was later adapted by Edna Foa and colleagues (1980) to include imaginal exposure and processing.

In Vivo Exposure

In vivo exposure involves exposure to feared stimuli in real life. It enables patients to confront stimuli and cues that trigger obsessive thoughts in a systematic manner with the support of their therapist. Stimuli are organized in a hierarchical fashion wherein patients are instructed to begin exposures to moderately distressing stimuli and work their way through progressively more distressing stimuli. It is important to note that effective exposures match the intensity of the obsession, meaning that treatment usually requires the patient to exceed the expectations of normal behavior (e.g., eating potato chips off a bathroom floor).

Imaginal Exposure

Imaginal exposure also triggers obsessions but in a different way. Instead of facing stimuli in real life, the patient is coached through imagining the details of their fears coming true. This technique enables people to play out the catastrophic outcomes that their OCD convinces them could happen if compulsions do not occur. This technique is particularly useful at targeting obsessions where in vivo exposure is either not logistically possible (e.g., burning in hell), safe (e.g., contracting HIV) or appropriate (e.g., molesting a child). Both types of exposure are most effective when performed in a repeated, prolonged manner (30–60 minutes) without engaging in any compulsions/rituals for up to two hours or until distress begins to dissipate (Foa, 2010).

Ritual Prevention

Ritual prevention requires the patient to abstain from performing compulsions/rituals that they believe either prevent a catastrophic outcome from occurring or reduce distress from an obsessive thought. Ritual prevention is encouraged after planned exposures in addition to day-to-day living (e.g., not using a shirt sleeve to open doors). This technique is vital in OCD treatment in that it facilitates corrective and inhibitory learning. Patients learn that (1) anxiety and distress naturally dissipate without compulsions and (2) their feared consequences are unlikely to occur in that even if the feared consequence does occur, it is almost never going to be as catastrophic as their OCD imagined and they can learn to tolerate the distress. Such learning enables patients to process the distress brought on by obsessions as opposed to instantly escaping it.

Processing

Processing occurs during and after exposures, and it involves a discussion about the patient's experience. Most of the conversation is about the degree to which the experience confirmed or disconfirmed the patient's expectation. The therapist asks questions related to the current level of distress and the desire to engage in a compulsion/ritual. Processing also involves more detailed discussion of the ways in which corrective and inhibitory learning occurred throughout episodes of exposure and ritual prevention. Such learning is ultimately what enables patients to develop a more adaptive relationship with their OCD and maintain long-term progress after treatment ends.

Family-Based CBT for Children

There has been a growing amount of literature (e.g., Marien et al., 2009; Storch et al., 2007) in support of increased family involvement in pediatric treatment of OCD. Prior to the development of family-based CBT (FB-CBT), parents did have some involvement in treatment, but at varying degrees based on the case. In FB-CBT, parents attend most (if not all) of the sessions, and siblings may be present as well. Generally speaking, the protocol includes psychoeducation about OCD and treatment; ideas regarding problem-solving, psychoeducation, and reduction techniques in respect of family accommodation; and ways to reinforce exposure completion/response prevention at home (Marien et al., 2009). Providers ideally want to teach parents and families how to be the best "coach" to the child with OCD. Many of the other tenets of ERP described in previous paragraphs apply here as well, with some modification in language and allowing for more space for parent coaching.

Empirical Support

Since its development in 1966, countless randomized controlled trials (RCTs), meta-analyses, and dissemination studies have examined ERP's utility in the treatment of OCD symptoms in adults and children (Eddy et al., 2004; Law & Boisseau, 2019; McKay et al., 2015; Olatunji et al., 2013; Reid et al., 2021). Only case studies have supported ERP's efficacy in older adults, as research on this population is generally sparse (Calamari & Cassidy, 1999; Carmin & Wiegartz, 2000). The earliest studies showed it to be superior to relaxation therapy, anxiety management, and waitlist (Rachman et al., 1971). Several investigations thereafter have additionally shown it to be efficacious across ages; in several countries, treatment settings, and levels of symptom intensity; and with diagnostic comorbidities (Abramowitz, 2006; Fals-Stewart et al., 1993; Freeston et al., 1997; Jones et al., 2012;

Lindsay et al., 1997; Storch et al., 2009). Specifically, Eddy and colleagues (2004) estimated that two-thirds of patients who received ERP saw improvements in symptoms, and roughly one-third were considered recovered. Reviews by Abramowitz (2006) and Foa and Kozak (1986) support earlier findings (Eddy et al., 2004), estimating that 50–60% of patients who receive ERP will show significant improvement with lasting results. ERP has also been shown to improve sleep, decrease depressive symptoms, and improve overall quality of life (Diefenbach et al., 2007; Storch et al., 2008, 2009). FB-CBT for children has shown to be effective in both individual and group formats. Results show remission rates for individual FB-CBT at 88% and 76% for group settings (Barrett et al., 2004). Further, 75% of youth in an intensive FB-CBT program and 50% of youth in a weekly FB-CBT program no longer met criteria for OCD upon completion of treatment (Storch et al., 2007). The degree of empirical support backing ERP's efficacy is why it is widely regarded as the psychological treatment of choice for OCD.

Despite the previously mentioned positive outcomes, ERP is not a flawless treatment that works for all cases of OCD and up to 30% of participants drop out of treatment prematurely (Abramowitz, 2006). A review by Middleton et al. (2019) highlighted issues with treatment adherence, poor insight, diagnostic comorbidities, and severity of OCD symptoms as primary indicators of poorer outcomes. ERP has been found to be less effective for those with repugnant obsessions (Garcia et al., 2010; Williams et al., 2013) and those whose compulsions are related to "just right" beliefs/sensations, as compared to feared outcomes (Foa et al., 1999). While research on comorbid depression is rather mixed, some research has suggested that severe depression (as opposed to depressive symptoms) predicts poorer outcomes (Abramowitz & Foa, 2000). Pinto et al. (2011) found that comorbid obsessive-compulsive personality disorder worsened ERP outcomes. Similarly, ERP was less beneficial for patients with comorbid autism spectrum disorder than for those without it (Flygare et al., 2020), and case studies have indicated that ERP is not suitable for those with psychotic disorders (Tundo & Necci, 2016).

Additional variables related to poorer outcomes include family members' adherence and therapist factors. High familial accommodation does in fact predict poorer ERP outcomes in children (Garcia et al., 2012; Storch et al., 2007). Additionally, Waters and Barrett (2000) theorize that OCD symptoms and family dysfunction operate in a cyclical manner. Patient nonadherence, specifically early homework incompletion and continued mental compulsions, is linked to poorer outcomes (Gillihan et al., 2012; Simpson et al., 2012; Wheaton et al., 2016). Lastly, therapists who encourage distraction during exposure, provide reassurance, and fail to treat core fears could produce poorer outcomes with greater relapse rates (Gillihan et al., 2012). There will be further explication of poorly executed exposures in Chapter 11.

CT

Theory

While there are several proposed models of CT for OCD, the model by Salkovskis (1985) is the best known. This model of OCD rests upon the theory that a person's emotional response to the disturbing and unpleasant nature of intrusive thoughts is largely due to faulty subjective appraisals whereby the person attaches significance and personal meaning to the intrusion. Cognitive theorists argue that dysfunctional beliefs about intrusive thoughts create and maintain OCD. Salkovskis' model also highlights how magnified beliefs of personal responsibility and power maintain OCD. People with OCD often believe that they have both the power and the responsibility to cause and prevent negative, sometimes catastrophic, outcomes. Application of CT techniques aims to address all of these problematic beliefs.

Treatment Description

Most of CT's protocol for OCD mirrors the protocols developed for depression and anxiety disorders. Therapists work collaboratively with patients to help them identify and re-evaluate the beliefs that lead to compulsions. Included techniques are psychoeducation, thought records, Socratic questioning, and behavioral experiments. While some of this cross-over with techniques used in manualized ERP, CT focuses much more on cognitive restructuring to alleviate suffering, whereas ERP is more concerned with behavior change. Most notably, CT does not require prolonged exposure and ritual prevention to reduce anxiety.

Cognitive Restructuring

Patients are instructed to write down their obsessions and associated interpretations in a thought record, along with what was happening right before the obsession occurred, the meaning attributed to the obsession, and the response to the obsession. The therapist then reviews the thought record with the patient and uses Socratic questioning to gently challenge the validity of their obsessions. The goal here is for patients to identify cognitive distortions.

Behavioral Experiments

Once the patient is skilled in identifying their obsessions and compulsions, the therapist will suggest behavioral experiments to further test and disprove the distortions of cause and effect, as it relates to the obsessive-compulsive cycle. Behavioral experiments typically occur outside of session as homework assignments and do not necessarily match the obsession's intensity. The results of such experiments typically spark further conversation about magical thinking and other distortions.

Empirical Support

CT specifically designed for OCD is newer than ERP and has been studied much less over the years. Beck and colleagues (1979) did, however, conduct trials that employed CT for OCD. The results showed a slight improvement with CT, but it is unclear how much of this was due solely to CT as it was used in combination with ERP. The impact of CT alone on outcomes is uncertain. When comparing CT to ERP, results have been mixed. Some research (i.e., McLean et al., 2001) has shown CT to be inferior to ERP, while other studies (i.e., Van Oppen et al., 1995) have shown it to be superior to ERP. Studies that define "efficacy" more conservatively favor ERP, while studies that define it as simply being asymptomatic show no significant difference (Fisher & Wells, 2005). Participants in both groups have shown significant improvement at one-year follow-up (Olatunji et al., 2013). While many studies show CT to be as efficacious as ERP, depressive symptoms improve faster with CT than with ERP (Cottraux et al., 2001). Consistent with the model proposed by Salkovskis (1985), CT is also most useful in targeting beliefs of responsibility, threat estimation, and over-importance of thoughts (Cottraux et al., 2001; van Oppen et al., 1995).

In Summary

OCD is a mental health condition characterized by repetitive thoughts and behaviors that interfere with a person's daily life and cause significant distress. Symptoms of OCD vary in intensity, duration, and insight, and it is primarily maintained by intolerance of uncertainty and poor distress tolerance. OCD has a strong link to suicidal thoughts and is often comorbid with other mental health conditions such as depression, EDs, and PTSD. ERP is a widely accepted treatment for OCD that involves facing and resisting obsessions and compulsions to reduce symptoms and suffering. CT has also been explored as a treatment for OCD, but its effectiveness is not yet clear. Some researchers have suggested that CT may be helpful when used before or in addition to ERP, but more research is needed before CT can be considered a first-line treatment for OCD.

Diagnostic Comorbidity and Phenomenological Overlap of Eating Disorders and Obsessive-Compulsive Disorder

As the Chapters 1 and 2 have highlighted, EDs and OCD impact people across the lifespan, with growing prevalence rates. Furthermore, numerous studies have shown that individuals with EDs have statistically higher rates of OCD and vice versa (Altman & Shankman, 2009; Angst et al., 2004; Bang et al., 2020; Kaye et al., 2004; Mandelli et al., 2020; Swinbourne & Touyz, 2007). Comorbid rates of OCD and EDs have been estimated to be anywhere from 20 to 60% (Godart et al. 2002, 2003; Halmi et al., 2005; Kaye et al., 2004; Speranza et al., 2001). Meta-analytic data shows that up to 44% of people with AN and 19% of people with BN have a secondary diagnosis of OCD, and 18% of people with an ED have a lifetime prevalence of comorbid OCD (Mandelli et al., 2020). Studies have also shown the presence of subclinical OCD symptoms in many restrictive ED presentations (Meier et al., 2020; Roberts, 2006). The relationship between anxiety disorders, OCD, and EDs is supported by genetic studies (Silberg & Bulik, 2005; Strober et al., 2007; Yilmaz et al., 2020). Childhood anxiety disorders and OCD have been linked to the onset of EDs (Erol et al., 2002; Swinbourne & Touyz, 2007). Many researchers have even proposed that OCD and EDs are part of the same spectrum of disorders (Bellodi et al., 2001; Neziroglu & Sandler, 2009; Pallister & Waller, 2008).

Individuals with OCD and AN exhibit a particularly complicated presentation that requires specific interventions and complex clinical expertise to yield positive treatment outcomes (Simpson et al., 2013; Storch et al., 2010). We can assume that malnutrition is the primary culprit leading to complications in this presentation, as it compromises medical safety, worsens cognitive functioning, hinders insight and perception of reality, and increases obsessionality (Keys, 1950). There is an argument by Strober (2004) that highlights "fear-learning" as a common denominator in anxiety and AN, wherein patients are more prone to respond to fear conditioning and quickly associate fear and weight gain after they begin to restrict. Steinglass and colleagues (2007) proposed that similar disturbances in the neural circuitry of people with OCD and AN lead to deficits in implicit learning, which in turn lead to rigidity, perfectionism, and an overall sense of being "stuck." This can cause avoidance of certain calories and "unsafe" foods, leading to weight loss. This weight loss may serve to maintain fears, but it also increases anxiety and causes negative consequences related to starvation, creating a self-defeating cycle. We will outline the overlapping presentations of OCD and EDs.

In an attempt to improve treatment outcomes for this population, we must first highlight the primary constructs that account for the phenomenological overlap and the differences between the two disorders. This chapter will briefly address the differences in the two disorders, followed by a review of what we believe to be the primary variables that account for the phenomenological overlap in this presentation. Primary variables discussed here include the following: (1) obsessionality/intrusive cognitions; (2) perfectionism; (3) avoidance; and (4) ritualistic behavior. We will also include some examples of comorbid presentations based on such variables. Lastly, we will briefly touch on the gap in treatment, and the implications of said gap.

Phenomenological Differences

Although there are more studies on the similarities between OCD and EDs with regard to behaviors, neurobiology, personality traits, and onset variables, there are notable differences in their psychopathology and clinical presentation (Jiménez-Murcia et al., 2007). For the purposes of this book, the differences highlighted here are exclusive to the variables we believe have the strongest implications for treatment outcomes. We specifically aim to improve clinicians' ability to successfully implement the currently identified empirically supported treatment for EDs and OCD.

Ego-Syntonic vs. Dystonic

A primary notable difference that researchers have identified is the ego-syntonic nature of most ED psychopathology compared to the ego-dystonic nature in which OCD typically presents (Sunday et al., 1995). This notion is consistent with Fairburn's transdiagnostic model for EDs, in that the overevaluation of body image and dietary restraint account for a disproportionate amount of self-worth and identity in individuals with EDs. We could argue that certain subtypes of OCD symptoms present as ego-syntonic in nature (e.g., obsessions and compulsions related to morality, self-image, etc.); however, the general consensus is that, by and large, symptoms are ego-dystonic for most OCD patients. This phenomenological trait engenders natural implications for treatment, specifically related to insight of illness, motivation for change, and compliance with recommendations for both disorders.

Cognitive and Physiological Implications

Another notable difference between the two disorders relates to the impact of psychopathology on cognitive functioning and medical stability. Eating pathology impacts the functioning of the brain and the body in a way that OCD typically does not. Individuals with EDs may require hospitalization or ongoing medical intervention in cases of severe symptomatology (e.g., low heart rate due to malnutrition or recurrent self-induced vomiting). This variable is most notable in cases of restrictive EDs (i.e., AN and ARFID) due to the effects of low body weight, chronic malnutrition, and nutritional deficiency. It is generally assumed that weight gain and increased nutritional intake must occur before any substantial cognitive change or emotional processing can successfully occur. Becker and colleagues (2020) also note that many individuals with BN are in a chronic state of semistarvation. This may not yield as many hospitalizations, but it could certainly impact cognitive functioning and insight.

Phenomenological Overlap

Obsessionality/Intrusive Cognitions

While data indicates some differences between OCD and EDs regarding the appraisals and control strategies of intrusions, both groups experience intrusive cognitions at a comparable frequency and emotional disturbance (García-Soriano et al., 2014). Similarly, individuals who are at high risk for developing an ED and OCD show greater frequency of obsessional thinking and eating-related intrusions than individuals with no risk of EDs and OCD (Belloch et al., 2016).

A differential analysis by García-Soriano and colleagues (2014) examined OCD-related intrusions in patients with OCD or an ED and found that intolerance of uncertainty in the OCD group and thought importance in the ED group predicted emotional disturbance and disruption. Individuals with EDs have also displayed equivalent or significantly higher scores than individuals with OCD on the Obsessive Beliefs Questionnaire, Interpretation of Intrusions Inventory, and Magical Ideation Scale (Lavender et al., 2006). Lastly, an analysis by Vanzhula and colleagues (2021) showed that the biggest connecting variable central to OCD and EDs was "difficulty controlling thoughts," meaning that intrusive thoughts in OCD cross over to worry and doubts about eating and body image in EDs.

Thought–Action Fusion

A specific type of cognitive distortion found in OCD was first described as thought–action fusion (TAF), wherein patients believed that having an obsessive thought was morally equivalent to acting on that obsessive thought (morality-TAF; Rachman, 1993). This original description was later adapted to the notion that intrusive thoughts can directly influence the probability of that thought coming to fruition (probability-TAF; Rachman & Shafran et al., 1999). Clinicians regularly see this phenomenon in OCD patients, and with repugnant obsessions in particular. Morality-TAF is also predictive of emotional disturbance in both OCD and EDs (García-Soriano et al., 2014). After Cooper et al. (1997) showed evidence of TAF occurring in those with EDs, Shafran and colleagues (1999) adapted the construct to "thought–shape fusion" (TSF) to better apply to the ED population.

Thought–Shape Fusion

TSF is broken down into three parts: (1) likelihood-TSF, (2) moral-TSF, and (3) feeling-TSF. Likelihood-TSF refers to the idea that simply thinking about eating a forbidden or "bad" food increases the likelihood that one's weight or shape will change. Moral-TSF mirrors morality-TAF but for forbidden foods. Feeling-TSF implies that having thoughts about forbidden foods increases the feelings of fatness. Results also indicated higher TAF-likelihood in Bulimia Nervosa Purging Type (BN-P) patients and lower TAF-moral in BED patients than healthy controls.

Shafran and Robinson (2004) later examined TSF more closely and confirmed its association in ED psychopathology. Results showed significantly more prevalent TSF in EDs compared to non-ED controls, which remained constant even when depression levels were controlled. Such findings suggest that TSF might be a direct expression of the overevaluation of eating behaviors, body weight, and body shape. We see this notion later reflected in Fairburn, Cooper, and Shafran's (2003) transdiagnostic model of EDs.

The transdiagnostic perspective on EDs was later supported by Roncero et al. (2011), who found higher obsessional beliefs in AN patients than in healthy controls, with BED patients scoring the most similar to healthy controls. Most clinicians treating patients with EDs would likely agree that their patients with AN tend to have higher degrees of obsessionality compared to their other ED patients. There are two important considerations related to the obsessionality seen in AN patients: (1) malnutrition and starvation is known to increase anxiety and obsessionality (Keys et al., 1950) and (2) obsessionality is perhaps what accounts for CBT-E's less than ideal outcomes in AN patients.

Perfectionism

Maladaptive perfectionism typically presents as a combination of self-evaluation with harsh self-criticism and unrelenting standards that are often inflexible, unreasonable, and leave no room for error (DiBartolo et al., 2008). Several studies have identified perfectionism as a variable involved in the onset and maintenance of OCD and EDs (Ashby & Bruner, 2005; Pollack & Forbush, 2013; Soreni et al., 2014; Wu & Cortesi, 2009). Given what we know about the psychopathology of both disorders as related to rules, rituals, and rigidity, perfectionism is a perfect fit as a correlating construct.

In a more classic presentation of perfectionism-infused OCD, a person may feel compelled to ensure that everything in his or her house is tidy and put away before leaving. The ritual involved in this presentation is likely rooted in the idea of things being "just right," and it may involve a fair amount of repetition. A common, yet lesser-known, face of perfectionism manifests as a person living in squalor because he/she cannot find the right time to clean the space to perfection. Perfectionism can present as a person proofreading an email several times before hitting send or as accidentally missing an important deadline on an assignment due to being unsatisfied with slight imperfections. Some individuals with OCD will go as far to say that they willfully choose to lose points on an assignment for lateness rather than subject themselves to the distress of tolerating imperfections.

Perfectionism is understood a bit differently in EDs. Researchers have identified it as a primary vulnerability trait in ED onset (Lilenfeld et al., 2006; Stice, 2002) and a common variable in ED maintenance (Fairburn, 2008; Shafran et al., 2004). With regard to onset, it is not uncommon for perfectionistic people to adopt the beliefs and behaviors that are typically associated with the "perfect diet" and the "perfect body." A patient who makes the decision to binge eat after having one cookie because "the day was already ruined" is a classic example of how clinicians see perfectionism manifest in ED maintenance. It is also believed that perfectionism is a primary variable that bridges the gap between OCD and EDs.

A review by Bardone-Cone and colleagues (2007) noted that the link between perfectionism and AN is long standing and widely accepted. However the link between perfectionism and BN is less clear. A common theme between perfectionism and BN relates to striving for a "perfect body" (Fairburn et al., 2003; Goldner et al., 2002). This domain of perfectionism often presents as one having unrelenting standards as regards eating behaviors and behaviors that impact body image. As a result of such standards, individuals with EDs often engage in food avoidance and exercise rituals in addition to other destructive behaviors believed to impact their body image (e.g., self-induced vomiting). There is also a fair amount of self-defeating dichotomy in their thinking and behavior (Lethbridge et al., 2011). It is not unusual for people with EDs to truly believe that the whole day has been tarnished from eating one cookie; this dichotomy in one's thinking also increases the risk of binge-eating.

Perfectionism usually results in a never-ending cycle of self-criticism, anxiety, guilt, and frustration, which of course has a negative impact on quality of life. In cases of EDs and OCD, perfectionism has the potential to seriously impair one's day-to-day functioning by leading to various types of self-defeating behavior. As intrusive cognitions are understood as unwanted, spontaneous, and discrete thoughts, images, and impulses that are difficult to control and interfere with activity (Clark, 2005), it comes as no surprise that individuals with OCD and EDs engage in a fair amount of avoidance.

Avoidance

While neither disorder truly begins with avoidance, it is perhaps one of the most notable maintenance variables in both disorders. In both OCD and EDs, avoidance is largely believed to occur in response to anticipation of feared outcomes and/or emotional distress (Becker et al., 2020; Clark, 2020; Waller & Mountford, 2015). Although OCD and EDs involve different feared content, patients with these disorders often engage in avoidance of feared stimuli and situations. In the case of OCD, avoidance may occur to prevent perceived harm to oneself or others (e.g., contracting or transmitting an illness). The idea of "harm" is usually intended to describe an undesirable effect on body weight, shape, and size.

The avoidance that commonly manifests in individuals with ED pertains to avoiding stimuli that provide information about their body, weight, shape, or size. Examples of this include avoiding weighing scales or not wearing form-fitting clothing. In the case of avoidance of form-fitting clothing, this functions to protect them against their own experience of their bodies in addition to the dreadful possibility of others negatively judging their bodies. Lastly – and perhaps the most obvious variable in ED maintenance that is not applicable to OCD – is the biological nature of eating behaviors as related to experiential avoidance. Persistent starvation and malnutrition often produce a state of alexithymia (Beadle et al., 2013), and binge-eating provides a rush of dopamine (Bello & Hajnal, 2010; Wang et al., 2011). Both of these states tend to produce a sense of emotional numbness that can certainly be appealing in the face of psychosocial stressors. When life circumstances require one to approach rather than avoid, individuals with OCD and EDs will likely engage in a fair amount of ritualistic behavior guided by rules and rigidity.

Ritualistic Behavior

Consistent with the literature on intrusive thoughts, perfectionism, and avoidance, the ritualistic behavior that we see in individuals with OCD and EDs is often motivated by maladaptive cognitions about catastrophic outcomes and firmly held beliefs about morality, achievement, and identity (Humphries et al., 2007). Therefore, most rituals function to alleviate or prevent the anxiety associated with such cognitive domains. Common examples of rituals seen in both disorders include reassurance seeking, checking, and ordering (Garner & Garfinkel, 1997; Humphries et al., 2007; Rachman & Hodgson, 1980). In both disorders, reassurance seeking often presents as either looking up information (e.g., Googling calories or signs of contracting HIV) or asking loved ones about behaviors related to fears (e.g., "Are you sure this won't make me gain weight?"; "You can't get HIV if you use a condom, right?"). Vanzhula and colleagues (2021) found that checking compulsions and rigidity around food are associated with restrictive eating, and hoarding behaviors are associated with binge-eating in clinical samples of EDs. A study by Pollack and Forbush (2013) supports the notion of a transdiagnostic model of comorbidity between OCD and EDs by highlighting a relationship between eating pathology, personality traits, and rituals in a community sample

With regard to the ritual of checking, we see increased body checking in individuals with stand-alone EDs and comorbid OCD. This behavior often presents as recurrent, excessive weighing, prolonged examinations of one's body in the mirror, and repeated grabbing and touching of various body parts. Several studies (e.g., Pretorius et al., 2012; Wang et al., 2019) have highlighted the role of cognitive rigidity as it relates to body dissatisfaction and checking behaviors in EDs. Individuals with AN in particular have difficulty with "big picture" thinking and mental flexibility (Wang et al., 2021). We see this phenomenon in OCD as well. For example, a person with OCD may fixate on one spot of dirt on a table rather than the room presentation as a whole and consequently have difficulty shifting one's focus away from that detail.

Rules and Rigidity

Individuals with OCD often have rules that they follow in their daily life and firmly held beliefs about the way they "must" behave. Conversely, individuals with EDs tend to have both rituals (for ED-related and non-ED-related domains) and overt rules that they follow regarding food and exercise. Such rules are typically informed by distortions related to the body's sensitivity to certain foods and exercise. It is also not uncommon for many people with EDs to subscribe to a belief of "the slippery slope," wherein isolated events of food indulgence or minimal breaks from exercise risk complete gluttony and laziness (e.g., "If I let myself eat a donut and discover that I like it, what if I want to get one every day?"; "If I take a week off of exercise on our trip to Jamaica, then I may lose all my progress and not want to get back in shape"). Thus, the rules function to prevent two primary feared outcomes: (1) weight gain/shape changes and (2) loss of control/overindulgence (Becker et al., 2020).

Examples of ED rules include having a list of permissible foods to eat on given days and times (e.g., "I don't eat carbs before dinner"; "I only eat one dessert food on Saturday nights"), an allotted calorie amount per day, and a detailed, excessive exercise routine. Such rules tend to be followed rigidly, with heightened emotional distress and cognitive inflexibility if something were to abruptly disrupt one's ability to follow the rules (e.g., an ankle injury that prevents running, a restaurant not having the salmon and steamed vegetable dish that one planned to order, etc.). When ample notice is given about a circumstance that prevents rule following, distress is typically managed by some form of behavioral compensation. This may include eating little to no food prior to the calorie-dense dinner, engaging in a purging behavior, or running extra mileage the following day.

Gap in Treatment

The overlap presents unique clinical challenges, and although there are empirically supported treatments for both disorders separately, there is currently little to no data on treatment outcomes nor a suggested treatment protocol for this comorbid presentation (Simpson et al., 2013). Moreover, empirically supported interventions for AN or BN may be contraindicated for effective treatment of OCD and vice versa. This is particularly problematic because ED studies have noted that comorbid OCD is associated with increased eating severity (Albert et al., 2001), longer duration of treatment (Milos et al., 2002), and poorer prognosis (Herpertz-Dahlmann et al., 2001; Val & Wade, 2015; Wentz et al., 2001).

The singular treatment study on comorbid EDs and OCD by Simpson and colleagues (2013) proposes the use of exposure-based CBT. This is further supported by the notion that exposure therapy is a suitable treatment for EDs (Becker et al., 2020; Waller, 2009). This gap in the literature has had a direct negative impact on both clinicians and patients alike. Well-trained specialists often face treatment-resistant outcomes and recurrent relapse in their patients, and patients in need of treatment struggle to find a treatment provider with competence in both disorders.

In Summary

EDs and OCD often co-occur, with studies showing that individuals with EDs have higher rates of OCD and vice versa. Subclinical OCD symptoms are often present in restrictive EDs and may impact treatment effectiveness and exacerbate symptoms. People with OCD and AN may have a particularly complicated presentation that requires specific interventions and clinical expertise for successful treatment. Malnutrition is believed to be a primary factor leading to complications in this presentation, as it can compromise medical safety, worsen cognitive functioning, hinder insight and perception of reality, and increase obsessionality. Primary variables that contribute to the overlap in presentation between OCD and EDs include intrusive cognitions, perfectionism, avoidance, and ritualistic behavior. There is a gap in treatment for this population that affects outcome.

Identifying Common Themes across Treatments for Eating Disorders and Obsessive-Compulsive Disorder

Although there is scant research on how to directly treat this comorbidity, there are robust evidence-based treatments for each disorder (discussed in Chapters 2 and 3) with positive outcomes. However, because there are a limited amount of dismantling studies, it is unclear which treatment features are necessary when providing the most effective and efficient therapy (Waller & Raykos, 2019). Knowing the most impactful mechanisms of action is especially important when we are suggesting a combined treatment for an existing comorbidity that does not currently have a manualized treatment available. This chapter will identify the common themes among the current evidenced-based treatments for each disorder, highlighting the shared therapeutic components and interventions. This identification will help understand which shared components may be responsible for change, which will be discussed in Chapter 6.

Similarities in ED Treatments

When broadly looking at the available empirically supported treatments for EDs, there are far more similarities than differences (Becker et al., 2020; Geller & Srikameswaran, 2015). Treatments including CBT-E, MANTRA, SSCM, Integrative Cognitive Affective Therapy (ICAT), Internet-based therapies, DBT, IPT, and FBT share many core tenets. All the aforementioned treatments include a collaborative framework, a motivational interviewing (MI) style, and relapse-prevention work. These therapies offer some type of psychoeducation, and most provide a clear rationale for how therapy will target mechanisms maintaining the disorders. While there are differences in technique execution, almost all the treatments provide skills for regulating affect, addressing the patient's value system, and examining relationships (Geller & Srikameswaran, 2015). IPT, DBT, and CBT-E address how a patient's self-worth affects symptoms, and both DBT and IPT intervene with interpersonal effectiveness skills directly (Champion & Power, 2012; Fairburn, 2008; Hagan & Walsh, 2021). Lastly, nearly all these treatments demonstrate an early behavioral change target around consistent eating, with an emphasis on weight gain for restrictive disorders, and many of them use in-session, visual collaborative weighing.

Exploring the Differences between CBT-E and FBT

When looking for commonalities between ED treatments, comparing CBT-E and FBT is a good place to start. These treatments have accumulated the most empirical evidence, with numerous studies testing their efficacy, and both have emerged as dominant with relevance to certain disorders and their associative presentations (i.e., diagnosis, duration of illness, age, support system variables, trauma, and motivation) (Fairburn et al., 2013; Kohn & Lock, 2015;

Lock et al., 2010; Lock & Le Grange, 2013; Wilfley et al., 2013). Despite these successes, the treatments themselves appear quite different at first glance.

Conceptualization

Most notably, the conceptualizations are different. In the FBT conceptualization, the disorder is externalized and the problem is viewed through a family systems paradigm wherein everyone works toward the solution. The child is seen as being unable to control their own choices around food. Because the child is starving and therefore likely experiencing cognitive deficits along with a preoccupation with body and food, their ability to make sound choices for their health are diminished (Keys et al., 1950). The first phase of treatment relies exclusively on the parent(s) or guardian(s) feeding the child every meal and snack. The externalization of the illness philosophy has its origins in narrative therapy as well as feminist theory (Madanes, 1981; White, 1986). This conceptualization contrasts with CBT, in which the problem is considered to be ego-syntonic, and which does not separate the person from the illness. In fact, CBT-E postulates that the core maintenance mechanisms of the ED involve patients overvaluing their shape, weight, and their ability to control them. This view puts the emphasis and the onus on the individual, further highlighting the contrast in conceptualization.

Family Involvement

Family involvement is essential to FBT, while in CBT-ED it is considered useful (especially with adolescents) but not central to treatment. In FBT, a therapeutic family meal occurs early in treatment. The therapist observes family dynamics that may help problem-solve resistance around meals and/or model noncritical language when the child is struggling. This intervention has its roots in structural family therapy and is not comparable to the goals of CBT-E (Minuchin, 1974). Additionally in FBT, the family is empowered to construct their own strategies for getting their child to eat. This instruction has its roots in Milan Systems Therapy (Selvini-Palazzoli, 1974). While the patient in CBT-E works with a therapist individually to learn how to better manage and control their behaviors (with some support from family in adolescent patients), FBT positions parents to have complete control over the child's eating behavior until closer to weight restoration.

Treatment Sequence and Logistics

In order to achieve success, FBT typically involves a multidisciplinary team that includes a primary therapist, a physician who ideally has specialized training in EDs, a nutritionist consultant, and a psychiatrist, if needed. Conversely, CBT-E typically relies heavily on one primary therapist, along with a physical assessment from a physician approving medical stability for outpatient care (as well as possibly throughout treatment if there are health concerns with increasing symptoms) and, when appropriate, a psychiatrist for medication management. FBT typically requires approximately 18 family sessions over a 6–12-month period, while CBT-E advises 20 individual sessions or 30–40 individual sessions for underweight patients (Lock & Le Grange, 2013). In the beginning stages of FBT, the single target is weight gain. All sessions in the first phase support this goal. Later sessions address adolescent autonomy and family issues that were put on hold early in treatment.

FBT does not directly address any of the same core mechanisms that CBT-E does, such as the overvaluation of shape, weight, mood/events affecting mood, or clinical features such as clinical perfectionism, mood intolerance, core low self-esteem, and interpersonal problems. CBT-E explores these mechanisms via the individual case formulation, without diving into any family systems work. This formulation yields protocols for behavioral change, directly addressing these mechanisms through various strategies (Dalle Grave et al., 2019).

Similarities between CBT-E and FBT

Early Essentials

Despite different conceptualization models and treatment-specific interventions, CBT-E and FBT have aspects wherein they may function in similar ways. Initially, both treatments begin by covering the same initial intervention targets (i.e., motivation, commitment, psychoeducation). Rather than focusing on the potential causes of the disorder, these treatments focus on maintenance mechanisms and adopt an "agnostic" view of the disorder. In both treatments, the therapist provides a great deal of psychoeducation and focuses on alliance building while underscoring the severity of the ED to increase motivation and commitment for change early in treatment (in FBT with parents and CBT-E with the individual). Both treatments involve providing a strong rationale for engaging in the treatment interventions with a clear call to action for change. They are both manualized and provide informed consent regarding typical outcomes, length of treatment, and expectations around structure in the first couple of sessions.

Behavioral Interventions

Both treatments employ behavioral procedures early in treatment that target healthy weight gain and/or a successful return to normal growth trajectories. For example, both treatments require in-session, collaborative weighing where the patient sees their weight. In each treatment, data from these weight exposures is used to inform food recommendations and monitor treatment progress. Both treatments use weight graphs to document weight changes and allow the patient and/or family to see progress and weight fluctuations.

Similarly, each treatment focuses on dietary restraint and restriction early in treatment. The CBT-E therapist utilizes psychoeducation, implements regular and consistent eating, uses self-monitoring records, and creates food hierarchies with the individual patient to directly target restraint and restriction. As referenced, the FBT therapist empowers parents to take control of food from their child (i.e., make all the meals, plate the meals) and provide them with enough nourishment for weight gain and restoration. Additionally, in FBT-BN (FBT for adolescent BN), the family is encouraged to bring in a "forbidden food" for the patient to eat during the family meal. After consuming the meal, they are instructed to have the patient spend time in the therapist's office to eliminate purging. Although this intervention is not explicitly set up as an exposure with ritual prevention, it certainly demonstrates a similar process. Thus, FBT may indirectly use exposure (a behavioral intervention) in a similar way to how CBT-E attempts to target dietary restraint and restriction. Food hierarchies in CBT-E, which resemble techniques typical to exposure therapy for anxiety disorders, are not directly targeted or structurally set up in FBT. However, if parents are feeding their child successfully, then the child may experience exposures indirectly. For example, a child will consume multiple meals and snacks and have exposure to a wide variety of foods, all while their parents prevent them from using compulsive behaviors such as purging or excessive exercise.

Additionally, FBT indirectly and CBT-E directly target body checking, body avoidance, and social comparison behaviors. For example, the patient may be asked to reduce the amount of time spent checking their weight/appearance and/or comparing their body to others by spending less time in front of the mirror, eliminating weighing themselves outside of appointments, reducing time spent on social media, focusing on their peer's faces instead of their bodies, etc. In CBT-E, patients who engage in body avoidance are often asked to wear more fitted clothes, eat in public, etc. Although there is no direct homework for body-focused behaviors in FBT, parents will often naturally encourage some of these interventions. For example, many parents hide the scale in their homes to avoid compulsive weighing. The FBT therapist also encourages the patient to increase peer support along with spending time with siblings after meals. This encouragement may decrease the amount of time spent on body image behaviors.

Value-Based Interventions

CBT-E directly addresses the value of shape, weight, and their control, which involves explicitly examining the patient's cognitions and values. CBT-E uses a pie chart later in treatment to illustrate the patient's overvaluation of appearance and food control in comparison to other areas of the patient's life that are undervalued or not valued at all. It also assists the patient in identifying their values and emphasizes alternative life domains to garner self-esteem. FBT does not address these clinical features directly; however, it strongly encourages peer social interaction, focuses on increased autonomy, and addresses age-appropriate problems in the last stage of treatment. Thus, FBT may also decrease the excessive value that these unhealthy domains have for the patient but in a more indirect way. Last, both treatments discuss and prepare for relapse-prevention and termination.

ED and OCD Treatment Similarities

When comparing the previously mentioned ED treatment to OCD treatments, there are many fundamental parallels. Broadly, treatment for OCD (i.e., ERP and CT) (Foa et al., 1997) include core themes that can be seen in nearly all evidence-based ED treatments: session agendas, providing structure and expectations for treatment, psychoeducation, a collaborative therapeutic relationship, and some level of self-monitoring.

As discussed in Chapter 4, individuals with both EDs and OCD commonly exhibit distress intolerance, uncertainty intolerance, perfectionism, avoidance, rigidity, and a tendency to overestimate the likelihood of feared outcomes (Salkovski et al., 2000; Waller & Mountford, 2015). These clinical features are targeted in treatment for both disorders. Given the importance of families in both FBT and FB-CBT for OCD, both treatments include parent training, accommodation reduction, and in-home interventions, thus highlighting many similarities. Although simply being exposed to a feared stimulus, such as food or a specific object, in FBT or CBT-E is not considered official exposure therapy, there may still be implicit effects that work to reduce the feared stimuli covertly, demonstrating similarities between treatments (Becker et al., 2020; Becker & Waller, 2017; Waller & Raykos, 2019). For example, a patient with an ED may be asked to reduce their exercise after self-monitoring documentation reveals an increase in exercise, which may serve as a safety (and compensatory) behavior to reduce anxiety about eating more food (or to prevent weight gain). This intervention may still help the patient receive corrective and inhibitory learning about weight and their ability to tolerate distress, despite the manual not explicitly framing this as exposure and ritual prevention.

Similarly, a parent regularly feeding their child in the beginning stages of FBT may ask the child to stay with them while they clean the kitchen or play a game with their siblings to reduce the chances of purging (which could be considered both compensatory and a prevention of a response). Although the specific mechanisms in FBT are unclear and eating in treatment is not necessarily set up like exposure, Hildebrandt and colleagues (2014) argue that FBT functions like family-assisted exposure because it provides a lot of exposure to the feared stimuli (eating large amounts of food frequently, seeing the weight on the scale weekly) along with tolerating the uncertainty of their final weight goal and using fewer safety behaviors (parents taking away exercise). Inadvertently, the child may have similar outcomes to ERP and learn corrective or inhibitory information (Becker et al., 2020). Furthermore, when patients are better nourished they will engage in typical exposures more willingly.

CBT-E uses hierarchies, along with targeting body checking and body avoidance, in a similar fashion to ERP. For example, early in treatment a patient may agree to eating more calories for breakfast, but in order to reduce anxiety, or in an effort to prevent any perceived judgment from others about her perceived changing body, they may choose to wear baggy clothes. This decision resembles a safety behavior. Given that the primary clinical goal is targeting weight gain and dietary restriction, patients are often told early in treatment to eat what feels comfortable, wear looser pants for comfort, have a plan for each meal, etc. (Fairburn, 2008). However, safety behaviors are challenged later in treatment. In stage three of CBT-E, the patient will create a hierarchy of feared foods and begin to practice eating foods that feel challenging, while also targeting safety behaviors (e.g., mirror avoidance), a method that looks very similar to aspects of OCD treatment.

Although it has been emphasized that exposure therapy accounts for most of the change in OCD treatment (Mclean et al., 2001), there is some evidence that CT may target maintenance variables in OCD that are not covered by behavioral interventions (Van Oppen et al., 1995). Similarly, although behavioral elements appear crucial in ED treatment, treatments such as CBT-E use elements similar to those seen in CT (i.e., reframing, behavioral experiments). In both CT for OCD and CBT-E for EDs, patients are asked to write down their thoughts after an activating situation, which is later reviewed in session. Both CBT-E and CT use psychoeducation about cognitive biases and accumulate evidence to challenge the validity of the patient's thoughts. A cognitive therapist may ask an OCD patient to run an experiment by reducing hand washing to test the associated improbable outcome (e.g., getting sick), and a CBT-E therapist may similarly ask a patient to test if abstaining from looking at their body in the mirror for a week will cause a five-pound weight gain. Both of these examples provide more opportunity to discuss distorted probability estimating, CT distortions, magical thinking, and other associated maladaptive beliefs.

In Summary

There is a lack of established treatment or treatment protocols for the overlap between EDs and OCD. Evidence-based treatments for each disorder have shown positive outcomes, but it is unclear which treatment features are necessary for the most effective and efficient therapy when treating comorbid EDs and OCD. This chapter identified common themes in current evidence-based treatments for each disorder and highlighted shared therapeutic components and interventions to better understand which shared components may be responsible for change. Overall, the most vigorous treatments for both OCD and EDs have similar components and cross-over interventions.

Identifying Mechanisms of Action across Treatments for Eating Disorders and Obsessive-Compulsive Disorder

As explored in previous chapters, there have been a number of studies that have established good efficacy and effectiveness for a range of psychological treatments for EDs as well as OCD, with treatments for the latter demonstrating more consensus in superiority. It is evident from our Chapter 5 review that these treatments have common therapeutic components and shared interventions. In looking at which components are the mechanisms of change across treatments for either disorder, exposure appears to be a key ingredient and primarily responsible for the effect in ERP for OCD. Overall, it is less clear how ED treatments are working. Because many of these treatments are presented as "treatment packages," it is difficult to identify which common factors are responsible for the reported outcomes (Murphy et al., 2009). Few studies have identified the most important mechanisms of change for patients with ED by dismantling treatment components, according to Waller and Raykos (2019).

Despite not fully understanding how these ED treatments actually work, it has been argued that the "active ingredients" across models are actually quite similar to one another (Becker et al., 2020). Chapter 5 highlighted common components across treatments including "starting well" essentials (i.e., psychoeducation, collaboration), elements of behavior therapy (i.e., exposure-based interventions), CT, interpersonal effectiveness, and value-based interventions. This chapter will use supporting empirical evidence to outline why these components may be the active ingredients and how they are working to make lasting change when treating EDs and OCD concurrently.

Early Essentials and Starting Well

Like most manualized treatments, the leading treatments for EDs and OCD include nonspecific, process-oriented therapy factors that are crucial to change early on in treatment. These factors include psychoeducation about symptoms, expectations for treatment, and nutritional information, as well as collaboration between the therapist and patient.

Psychoeducation

Given that psychoeducation has been demonstrated as an effective stand-alone treatment in some disorders, such as depression and anxiety (Brown & Lewinsohn, 1984; Donker et al., 2009), we propose that it is crucial for this comorbidity as well. Although few studies have investigated the effectiveness of psychoeducation in ED treatment, data suggests this variable is a direct mechanism of action. An early study by Olmstead et al. (1991) examined the impact of a brief psychoeducational group (EG) compared to standard CBT with BN patients. The individual CBT group was found to be superior to the EG only for patients with a more intense ED presentation (e.g., vomiting more than 42 times a month prior to treatment, etc.). This suggests that psychoeducation may have assisted in symptom reduction for those using symptoms less frequently, making it a possible mechanism of action in treatment (Olmstead et al., 1991).

There are no studies specifically examining the impact of psychoeducation on the treatment of OCD. However, psychoeducation is an important aspect of both ERP and CT. Psychoeducation helps to explain the reasoning behind the techniques used in treatment and provides patients with an understanding of why they are being asked to change their thinking and/or behavior. Many individuals with OCD view their intrusive thoughts negatively, which leads them to employ avoidance or use compulsions. This avoidance behavior prevents inhibitory learning, hinders the development of distress tolerance, and increases the likelihood that the thoughts will return, thus creating a vicious cycle. Psychoeducation that focuses on challenging negative appraisals, self-criticism, thought–action fusion, and normalizing intrusive thoughts is essential for breaking this cycle.

Collaboration

Providing education about OCD and its treatment not only helps to explain the rationale for treatment, it also enhances the therapeutic process by fostering collaboration between patient and therapist. According to Abramowitz (2013), it is important for both the therapist and the patient to have a clear understanding of the theory behind exposure therapy in order to achieve optimal treatment outcomes. This shared knowledge allows the therapist and patient to work together to identify and address covert rituals or mental compulsions that may hinder progress if not detected. Because behavioral interventions (i.e., exposure) can be difficult for patients and may lead to drop out, creating a safe and supportive environment through collaboration can be crucial.

Similarly, research has consistently shown that patients and providers prefer a collaborative stance (Geller et al., 2009; Geller & Dunn, 2011) during ED treatment as well. It could be argued that collaboration and other nonspecific factors, such as unconditional positive regard, are particularly important in the treatment of EDs due to their ego-syntonic nature and the accompanying shame that many individuals experience regarding their ED behaviors. Some individuals with EDs may identify closely with their disorder and resist changes to their identity, which can be aversive. A collaborative stance, in which the therapist and patient work together toward treatment goals, can be crucial in helping these individuals to make the necessary shifts in their identity and behavior in order to achieve lasting change.

Therapists treating OCD and EDs need to provide a compelling rationale for their patients to engage in behaviors that may cause fear or anxiety, such as touching a dirty floor or eating dessert. They can do this through the use of psychoeducation and by creating a collaborative environment that promotes strong and early change in treatment. Many studies have found that achieving early engagement and behavior change in ED treatment, such as ceasing purging by week 4 or gaining 2.4 kg in the first 5 weeks, is associated with better treatment outcomes (Fairburn et al., 2004, 2009; Le Grange et al., 2008). Early change also appears to be a robust predictor of eventual treatment outcomes in OCD, further highlighting overlap (da Conceição Costa et al., 2013). This emphasizes the importance of starting treatment well and engaging patients early on in order to achieve optimal results.

Behavior Therapy

Most empirically based treatments for OCD and EDs utilize behavioral interventions as a way to reduce symptoms. In OCD treatment, these behavioral interventions are directly presented as exposure in ERP and behavioral experiments in CT. In ED treatment, behavioral strategies are common, but are often presented less directly and are integrated with other elements. As Chapter 5 pointed out, examples of behavioral strategies within CBT-E and FBT include targeting dietary restraint and restriction, collaborative weighing, and use of weight graphs. The following sections highlight the empirical evidence for using behavioral therapy (BT) with this comorbidity, as well as providing a more in-depth look at why BT works for these disorders.

Empirical Evidence

There is a stronger evidence base and general consensus for the use of BT as a mechanism of action in the treatment of anxiety and OCD compared to EDs (Parker et al., 2018; Tolin, 2009; Waller & Raykos, 2019). Although there are fewer studies and less research on the mechanisms of action for ED treatments, it has been argued that behavioral components are important in these treatments and may account for a significant portion of the change that occurs during treatment (Becker et al., 2020; Waller & Raykos, 2019). In studies that have attempted to identify the specific components of ED treatments that are most responsible for change, behavioral interventions have often emerged as key. For example, one study found that BT had the lowest drop-out rate, the quickest symptom reduction, and was more effective than CBT when compared to CBT and supportive group therapy for BN (Freeman et al., 1988). Another study found that 71% of participants in the ERP group ceased bingeing and purging (Wilson et al., 1986) These findings suggest that behavioral interventions may be particularly effective in the treatment of EDs.

Another behavioral technique that has shown promising results in the treatment of EDs is cue exposure (Jansen et al., 1989), which is based on the principles of classical conditioning. It aims to reduce the association between a conditioned stimulus (e.g., watching TV) and an unconditioned response (e.g., binge eating) by repeatedly exposing the individual to the stimulus in a controlled environment with gradual exposure. In a study by Bulik and colleagues (1998), cue exposure was compared to relaxation training after patients completed CBT for BN. The patients in the cue-exposure treatment group experienced a reduction in symptoms (i.e., dietary restraint, purging, body image dissatisfaction, anxiety related to binge cues). This reduction in symptoms was maintained at a three-year follow-up (Carter et al., 2003; McIntosh et al., 2011). These preliminary results suggest that cue exposure may be a useful technique in the treatment of EDs.

Regarding the impact of behavioral interventions in adult AN, a small but influential study ($N = 8$) by Channon et al. (1989) compared CBT to BT for AN. BT included a combined approach of graded exposure to fear foods and relaxation techniques. While both groups showed some improvement, no significant differences were found. Channon et al. (1989) noted that cognitive elements of CBT may not add to the treatment for AN. More recently, a case series by Steinglass et al. (2012) developed a brief, 12-session treatment wherein ERP (based on the Foa & Kozak [1986] manual) was applied to recently weight-restored adult AN patients during inpatient treatment. The results included a decrease in fear around eating evidenced by an overall increase in caloric intake.

These studies demonstrate that behavioral techniques are key mechanisms of action and are at least partially responsible for the outcomes revealed. It is well documented that the most successful treatments for anxiety disorders and OCD include behavioral components (Hans & Hiller, 2013), namely exposure-based techniques (Kaczkurkin & Foa 2015). Considering the empirical evidence, along with the phenomenological overlap between EDs and OCD discussed in Chapter 4, it is reasonable to conclude that behavioral techniques are integral to all efficacious ED treatment (Becker et al., 2020). Understanding the nuances of these interventions and how they work may shed light on how they can be enhanced and applied to this relatively nonunderstood comorbidity.

Exposure Theory

Exposure therapy is a powerful BT that is used effectively in the treatment of both OCD and EDs. It is unclear exactly how exposure therapy produces its effects (Hofmann, 2008), and it may work differently for different individuals (Craske et al., 2014). For example, when providing weight exposures, some patients complete treatment without any distress or fear when stepping on the scale. Other patients end treatment still reporting some distress, but are no longer bothered by the distress and it does not affect their behavior. Given that recent research on OCD indicates that the two leading theoretical frameworks – emotional processing theory (i.e., habituation model; Foa & Kozak, 1986) and inhibitory learning theory (Craske et al., 2008) – may both be separate, unique change mechanisms (Elsner et al., 2022), it is possible that exposure to the scale worked differently for these groups of people

Emotional Processing Theory (EPT)

The goal of exposure through the lens of EPT is for anxiety to be reduced. This is achieved by structuring repeated contact with a feared stimulus while eliminating avoidance, safety, or escape behaviors, or any other rituals. Over time, exposure to a nonthreatening feared stimulus will eventually lead to a natural reduction in fear, thus illustrating that habituation has occurred (Benito & Walther, 2015). EPT has historically been considered the underlying framework for understanding exposure therapy and the process of habituation (Barlow, 2004; Foa & Kozak, 1986; Kaczkurkin & Foa, 2015). This theory posits that fear is represented in the brain by associative networks or cognitive fear structures (Kaczkurkin & Foa, 2015; Lang et al., 1971). This stored fear information becomes activated when the person encounters the feared stimuli or something that resembles it (Kaczkurkin & Foa, 2015). For example, Gary once believed dogs were safe but then had an experience where he was bitten by an off-leash, frightened dog. This experience consequently resulted in a fear of all dogs. According to EPT, it is assumed that his fear structure of dogs has changed. Gary now has a fear response to dogs and stimuli associated with dogs, which becomes activated even in an objectively safe situation. Walking past the gated dog park near his work activates so much fear that he now runs past it. Gary's reactions do not correspond to the level of actual danger walking past a gated dog park should evoke. Gary uses safety behaviors (runs past dogs) and avoidance (finds a different work route) to reduce the chances of an (improbable) attack, as well as the anxiety associated with this outcome. These avoidance efforts and safety behaviors provide short-term relief that is very reinforcing but which ultimately prevents new, safe experiences with dogs, thereby preventing new learning and maintaining the fear.

In EDs, a similar process occurs in relation to eating and weight-related fears. For example, Kenya noticed her weight was higher when she checked on the scale. She attributed this weight increase to a dessert she had the night before. This experience resulted in an erroneous belief that if she eats even one dessert, she will gain five pounds. In order to avoid weight gain and the subsequent negative emotions, she has not eaten a dessert in years (avoidance). When her parents try to persuade her to eat a dessert, she states the only way she would be able to do so is if it is sugar free (safety behavior).

EPT hypothesizes that exposure works by way of habituation, where the fear structures will be modified when they are activated and faced with incompatible information. This habituation can occur during a single trial of exposure (i.e., within-session habituation) and across trials (i.e., between session habituation) (Rauch & Foa, 2006). For Gary, this would indicate that exposure to dogs without any safety behaviors while observing no dog attacks, or, for Kenya, eating a dessert regularly while eliminating safety behaviors and not observing large changes in weight overtime, will reduce their fear responses to the respective feared stimuli. With the help of incompatible information modifying the fear structure when a person is exposed to the stimuli, in the absence of safety behaviors and rituals, the fear reaction is expected to decrease – and habituation is said to have occurred (Kaczkurkin & Foa, 2015).

Inhibitory Learning Theory (ILT)

The second theory, ILT, offers a different approach to understanding and executing exposure therapy. This theory suggests that the brain cannot unlearn fears stored in memory. ILT explains that exposures create new, nonthreatening associations (that become memories) which encourage extinction learning (Craske et al., 2014). For example, as Gary was attacked and bitten by a dog, dog stimuli are now conditioned to elicit a fearful response. In other words, Gary learned that dogs are scary. ILT postulates that Gary's brain may never erase that memory of when a dog was scary and harmful. However, by having many more new, neutral, or positive experiences with dogs (through repeated exposure), his brain will have an easier time retrieving nonfearful memories. In other words, these novel associations with dogs inhibit his brain's retrieval of the "old" fearful memories or associations. This leads to a more neutral reaction toward dogs, which will increase motivation to walk past the dog park or hang at his friend's house, thus developing additional neutral memories and eventually extinguishing the phobia. To put simply, repeated exposures work by diluting the original memory wherein the fear was learned.

This is different from EPT, which postulates that exposure modifies fear structures and changes the actual beliefs of the feared stimulus through new experiences. ILT hypothesizes that more neutral-associative experiences gained through exposure allows for easier retrieval of a neutral memory. In utilizing exposure through ILT, anxiety reduction in the short-term is less emphasized. Instead, the focus is on optimizing safety learning. If the new memories are numerous and strong, it will be harder for the old fear-based memory to compete with the new, robust positive or neutral memories (or inhibit the danger meaning). Violating expectancies (i.e., targeting the patient's assumptions), is one way to create stronger learning and therefore enhance extinction. For Gary, he may expect that any dog will attack him (e.g., growl and bite at him). In Kenya's case, she may assume eating any portion of a dessert (e.g., half of a cupcake) will cause immediate weight gain of up to three pounds or that she won't be able to handle the after-effects (e.g., feelings of guilt that distract her all day and thus make her unable to complete any work). Through exposure, patients often find that their expectations about either the feared stimuli (the dog attacked) or their reactions to the feared stimuli (upset all day or could not get out of bed) will not come true. Highlighting their assumptions and then using exposures to violate these expectancies is especially important for people with EDs where part of the pathology includes a "broken cognition" or an exaggerated correlation between how food affects weight (Fairburn, 2013; Waller & Mountford, 2015). There are additional strategies to help strengthen safety learning, such as varying the types of exposure (e.g., different types of dogs or different types of desserts) and where exposure occurs (e.g., eating dessert at a restaurant or after making it at home), and layering exposures (e.g., using imaginal exposure with in vivo exposures), as well as targeting distress tolerance (versus the reduction of anxiety) during exposures (Becker et al., 2020; Craske et al., 2008; Hofmann, 2008).

There are arguments for conducting exposure within the framework of both EPT and ILT, and a recent study suggests that both processes (i.e., habituation, distress-related expectancy violation) contribute to outcomes during exposure therapy independently (Elsner et al., 2022). Targeting anxiety levels through habituation can be useful when there is an exaggerated, anxious reaction to neutral situations that impedes the patient's life. It can also be clinically relevant to target anxiety levels because a patient may be more resistant or even drop out of treatment if their anxiety levels are not targeted or reduced (McGuire & Storch, 2019). However, exposure within ILT does not focus on reducing the feelings of anxiety; instead, the emphasis is on the critical ingredient of building distress tolerance (Craske et al., 2014). The objective of building up tolerance to anxiety instead of aiming to reduce anxiety can be especially powerful – a skill that can be applied to both ED and OCD patients (see Chapter 10 for the importance of distress tolerance). Both populations often have a belief that anxiety is intolerable, which can maintain the illness and may influence expectations around exposures (i.e., "this exposure therapy will eliminate my anxiety"). Framing exposures through a distress- tolerance lens can help patients understand that they need to strengthen their "muscles" for distress (e.g., anxiety, uncertainty) instead of trying to completely eliminate these feelings.

BT and Malnourishment

In addition to the learning models explaining why BT (e.g., exposure) is an effective treatment for OCD and EDs, BT may also work for EDs specifically because dietary restriction is targeted via caloric increase, weight gain, and incorporating a variety of foods. Attempts to avoid food or limit overall intake often lead to malnourishment and result in reduced cognitive functioning and other psychological consequences (e.g., obsessionality, rigidity). Zandian et al. (2007) argue that the effect of malnutrition, as a consequence of starvation, accounts almost entirely for the presentation of EDs. This is bolstered by numerous studies that indicated that early weight gain and/or regulated eating are associated with optimal recovery outcomes (Doyle et al., 2010, Hartmann et al., 2007; Le Grange et al., 2014; Lock et al., 2006; Madden et al., 2015) and an immediate reduction in psychiatric symptoms (Wilson et al., 2002). Even nonunderweight patients can be affected by restriction. Nisbett (1972) highlighted that higher weight individuals tend to undereat or maintain a weight that is too low for their set point given the pressures of society and the misunderstanding of the causes of obesity. This underscores the importance of targeting restraint and restriction for all EDs during treatment. Such effects are elaborated further in Chapter 7.

Overall, these results underscore that direct intervention on starvation is a key mechanism of action. Patients with a comorbid OCD diagnosis are also likely to experience an exacerbation of their obsessive thinking due to starvation effects, which makes these interventions so crucial to treatment. Given how significant dietary restriction is to the individual's health and how this malnourishment can maintain their illness, behavioral interventions (e.g., self-monitoring records, exposure) that directly target dietary restraint and restriction are crucial. Overall, BT may also work for patients with EDs because it helps increase food intake, thereby reducing the malnourishment that causes and prolongs psychological effects.

Cognitive, Interpersonal, and Value-Based Therapies

Despite BT appearing very necessary to anxiety and OCD treatment, and very likely integral to effective ED treatments, behavioral components alone in ED treatment (unlike OCD treatment) do not appear sufficient to achieve optimal outcomes for recovery (Waller & Raykos, 2019). The following two sections highlight the limitations of behavioral therapies for EDs and the possible advantages of drawing from alternative interventions including cognitive, interpersonal, and value-based therapies for the treatment of this comorbidity.

Empirical Evidence

Some early studies attempted to dismantle treatment features to understand what is working in ED treatment. There are additional studies indicating that BT alone is not sufficient for remission. For example, Agras et al. (1989) investigated the most optimal therapeutic components for BN and found that BT was not enough. More specifically, Agras et al. found that adding response prevention (RP) of self-induced vomiting did not enhance CBT. The authors even noted that a possible "deleterious effect" occurred wherein the additional RP intervention appeared to reduce the efficacy of the CBT package.

Another early study by Wilson et al. (1991) found that BT alone was insufficient for BN treatment, as CBT with ERP did not show improved effectiveness over CBT alone. In a comparison of BT, CBT, and IPT by Fairburn et al. (1993), BT, defined as regaining control over eating, establishing a regular eating pattern, and ending dieting, was found to be less effective than CBT and IPT. The study showed high attrition in BT treatment, and only a few patients fully eliminated bingeing and purging. Although these findings do not definitively determine the elements responsible for change, they suggest that CT and interpersonal elements play a role in treatment success. Currently, no evidence exists that CBT is more effective than IPT for BED treatment, as IPT has proven effective in reducing binge eating and related thoughts (Fairburn et al., 1993; Karam et al., 2019; Wilfley et al., 1993, 2002; Wilson et al., 2010). IPT focuses only on the patient's interpersonal experience and doesn't address behavioral factors or utilize behavioral interventions, unlike CBT. Further, both DBT and CBT-E have interpersonal effectiveness modules, suggesting that interpersonal interventions may play a key role in treatment success (Hagan & Walsh, 2021). These findings indicate that therapy ingredients other than behavioral interventions may contribute to optimal results (for BN and BED), as IPT is not a BT.

In viewing treatment outcomes for AN, FBT has demonstrated the most success in adolescents. Although we have previously argued that (indirect, family-assisted) exposure is likely an active ingredient, it should still be noted that the phase three targets (i.e., providing support for adolescent issues and development) may possibly account for some of the treatment success. Because there is not a superior treatment for adult AN, it is difficult to identify the most active components. It is possible that the effects of malnourishment and low body weight may perhaps be a reason why the cognitive elements of CBT do not necessarily enhance outcomes for AN. Channon et al. (1989) found that both groups showed some improvement without significant differences. Additionally, because SSCM has demonstrated some basis of evidence for adult AN treatment, it is possible that nonbehavioral elements (e.g., psychoeducation, motivation, strong therapeutic alliance, and individual preferences/differences) could account for the treatment success (Waller & Raykos, 2019).

Theory

Despite ample evidence that early essentials such as psychoeducation, clear treatment expectations, and collaboration, and BT techniques such as exposure, play important roles in treating both OCD and EDs, these components alone may not lead to optimal outcomes and full remission for EDs. To achieve optimal results, it's crucial to include additional effective treatment components like CT, interpersonal effectiveness training, and value-based interventions.

CT

CT was first advanced by Aaron Beck for depression and is a widely used treatment for a number of disorders, as Chapter 3 highlighted. This tri-part model explains that thoughts, feelings, and behaviors are interrelated. Through a collaborative process of identifying these patterns between the therapist and the patient, CT targets maladaptive and distorted thinking through a number of techniques (e.g., examining evidence for and against the thoughts, empirical hypothesis-testing, reframing thoughts). In this process, the unhelpful cognition is identified, the validity examined, and the patient is encouraged to develop a more accurate thought which will elicit more positive emotions and adaptive behaviors.

In CBT-E, thoughts about food, weight, shape, and the patient's interactions in the world are all targeted. For example, Ava records in her self-monitoring log that she has eaten a bagel and then writes, "I am out of control and lazy for choosing a bagel." By collaboratively developing a definition of lazy or being out of control with Ava, and then examining the validity for those definitions, Ava can begin to reframe her thoughts and develop more adaptive ways of thinking about food and eating. Consequently, Ava may feel reduced distress and increased motivation to eat bagels once bagels are no longer associated with laziness.

IPT

Although there remain gaps in the current literature regarding how or why IPT works, Murphy and colleagues (2009) attribute the reduction in ED symptoms in IPT to the increases of self-efficacy and self-esteem resulting from a decrease of interpersonal problems targeted in treatment. They found that the increase in self-efficacy and self-esteem may take some time to shift, which may account for IPT's delayed but similar results for BN compared to CBT. By reducing interpersonal problems and improving a person's overall quality of life, self-efficacy in making friends and problem-solving in relationships increases, leading to higher self-esteem, less distress, and healthier coping mechanisms. This may be the mechanism of action in IPT, which leads to increased self-esteem.

Value-Based Interventions

Although interpersonal effectiveness is not a primary target in CBT-E and treatments are very different from one another, it is partially possible that CBT-E and IPT are both effective because they both increase self-esteem. Self-esteem is often based on what people value, such as appearance. For patients with EDs, appearance is often the main contingency from which they evaluate themselves. Due to the nature of EDs, especially given their ego-syntonic nature, there is a strong connection between self-esteem and shape or weight. Interventions in therapy (i.e., the pie chart in CBT-E) that target these self-esteem contingencies and shift values may contribute to a reduction in ED symptoms. Self-esteem and self-efficacy are primary mechanisms of action for IPT and integral to treatment. In FBT, there may be less focus on this, but phase three interventions may also target values or ways to increase self-esteem and be a mechanism of action within FBT.

In Summary

Overall, while there is limited research on the treatment of co-occurring OCD and EDs, there are several effective treatments available. Dismantling studies have shown that BT, particularly exposure-based interventions, is a key component in the treatment of OCD. For EDs, the active ingredients across treatment models are similar and may include elements of BT, psychoeducation, collaboration, CT, interpersonal effectiveness, and value-based interventions. These additional components may be less important for OCD but should not be overlooked when treating both disorders together. It is important to consider all these elements when developing treatment plans for individuals with co-occurring OCD and EDs.

This section of the book aims to identify what we have found to be the most common pitfalls and barriers that clinicians face when treating patients with both disorders. We will highlight the problematic reality of limited treatment providers with expertise in both disorders, and thus who are more likely to fall into one or more of these pitfalls. We will also include theoretical underpinnings and empirical findings where applicable to support why it is plausible to assume that the available manuals for each disorder are insufficient for sidestepping these pitfalls. This section also functions to preface Section III of the book, which will focus on tips and suggestions to better navigate the complexities of this comorbidity.

Underweight and Malnourished Patients

It is no secret that individuals who are underweight and/or malnourished present to treatment with unique challenges and considerations that need to be addressed for successful treatment of this comorbidity. It is important to note that underweight refers to a weight that is below where one's body would be at homeostasis. Additionally, individuals with higher weights may still be malnourished and experiencing nutritional deficiencies. There are several reasons, both psychological and medical, to account for being malnourished. Restrictive EDs (i.e., AN, ARFID, and ON) are characterized by the intentional limitation of food intake, which leads to developmental weight changes and health implications. Individuals with chronic anxiety disorders such as generalized anxiety disorder GAD and OCD may experience unintentional weight loss and malnutrition due to decreased appetite or nausea (Hofer & Schelling, 2001; Roelofs et al., 2008). These presentations have implications for symptom presentation, treatment course, and outcomes.

Low body weight and malnourishment are dangerous consequences of restrictive EDs (i.e., AN, ARFID, and ON) and anxiety-based disorders like GAD and OCD, and they have notable implications for treatment. EDs are unique among psychiatric disorders in that their symptoms impact the whole body and organ system. Prolonged malnutrition leads to extreme weight loss and negatively impacts brain and organ functioning. Current weight fluctuations and weight history are often of primary concern in patients with a clear presentation of an ED, whereas low weight may go unnoticed or be normalized in patients with an anxiety-based presentation. Patients with a primary ED expect to discuss weight, while patients with a primary anxiety disorder may be surprised and confused to do so. Regardless of the presentation, underweight and malnourished patients may be hesitant or resistant to treatment recommendations that involve weight gain and increased food intake.

This chapter discusses the definition and implications of being underweight, the effects of underweight and malnourishment on the body's organ systems, the importance of medical care in treatment, the effects of starvation on symptom presentation and treatment planning, and dietary considerations for weight restoration. It also considers the efficacy of exposure therapy in the case of co-occurring EDs and OCD.

Operationalizing "Underweight"

Although AN is more commonly associated with the subsequent psychological effects of malnourishment, restricting intake can lead to similar effects even in nonunderweight individuals. Nisbett (1972) highlights that higher weight individuals often undereat because of (1) misleading assumptions that obesity is a result of diet despite much evidence implicating other variables (e.g., genetics, polycystic ovary syndrome, food deserts) and (2) societal pressures to be thin. Nisbett argues that these pressures and assumptions may result in a person being underweight for their genetic weight set point regardless of whether they meet the criteria for classification as "overweight" or "obese" (i.e., BMI). Nisbett (1972) further identifies striking parallels between "obese" individuals and underweight individuals (e.g., eating behaviors, emotionality), suggesting that hunger is a shared factor. There are also a number of recent studies (e.g., Accuso et al., 2016; Berner et al., 2013; Bodell & Keel, 2015; Bodell et al., 2016; Butryn et al., 2006; Lowe et al., 2011) suggesting that patients exhibiting weight suppression effects, regardless of presenting BMI, still likely need to gain weight for their ED cognitions to subside. Current ED treatment programs have shifted to consider all patients as having malnutrition effects due to their illness, regardless of presenting BMI (Peebles et al., 2017).

Despite conventional wisdom that a BMI below 18.5 is associated with the stereotype of a frail and gaunt appearance, it is not the only indicator of underweight and malnourishment. It is also possible for individuals to be underweight or malnourished with a BMI within the "healthy" or "overweight" range, and, as a result, these individuals may not be flagged for possible EDs or malnourishment. Additionally, pediatricians may be more likely to screen for lipid abnormalities and insulin resistance rather than EDs in youth with higher BMIs, which can further contribute to the lack of diagnosis and treatment for underweight and malnourished individuals (Peebles & Sieke, 2019).

Why do we have a skewed picture about what it means to be underweight? Some include the widespread reliance on BMI in the medical community (despite flaws), the misunderstanding or overattribution of lifestyle and weight, along with the media representation of body image, weight, and health. It is not uncommon for physicians to gloss over patient weights that are considered mildly underweight, attributing the low weight to athletics or a fast metabolism. This same degree of "grace" is often not given for individuals who are considered mildly "overweight." In many of these cases, exercise or dietary changes are encouraged without even inquiring about the person's baseline diet and exercise regimen, or consideration of their genetics or relevant biological factors (e.g., a diagnosis of polycystic ovary syndrome [Hoeger et al., 2016] or whether their mother had gestational diabetes, which is correlated with higher body weight [Lawlor et al., 2008]). Put simply, weight bias is largely responsible for this problematic oversight (Peebles & Sieke, 2019). Failure to identify restrictive EDs early in the disorder's onset often means that windows for vital intervention may have already closed by the time a diagnosis is made. This unfortunate, yet common, clinical oversight has implications for symptom progression, treatment planning, and overall prognosis (Puhl et al., 2013). In the case of comorbid OCD, the patients' obsessionality is likely to worsen over time due to continued starvation and weight loss, complicating the treatment plan.

Atypical AN

The DSM-5's diagnostic criteria for AN no longer includes the rigid numerical threshold for weight (i.e., 15% under ideal body weight) that prior editions included. Despite this change, there is still an emphasis on weight that falls under the "normal" range per what is expected within the context of age, sex, developmental trajectory, and physical health (APA, 2013).

Severity of the presentation is based on BMI. Individuals falling within a "normal" or higher weight range will not meet the criteria for AN. Instead, these individuals would be considered as presenting with atypical AN despite engaging in intense restriction and/or falling under their healthy set point but not low enough to be considered in the AN category. This presentation of restrictive eating currently falls under the OSFED diagnosis.

Regardless of diagnostic criteria, the presentation of atypical AN is almost identical to typical AN (APA, 2013). There is no substantial difference in obsessions for those with typical AN and atypical AN (Levinson et al., 2019). Patients engage in the same extreme food restriction that typically leads to notable malnutrition, consistently engage in behaviors that prevent weight gain, and psychologically experience the same cognitions (i.e., an intense fear of gaining weight or "becoming fat," a disturbance of body image perception, self-evaluation unduly influenced by body image). It is important to note that they may or may not lose rapid weight (Keski-Rahkonen et al., 2007) regardless of intense restriction. The only factor that precludes a diagnosis of AN is that their weight is within or above the "normal" range (APA, 2013). Typically, these individuals simply have not reached the BMI threshold of "underweight" due to one of two reasons: (1) they had a higher premorbid BMI before restriction began and/or (2) they have a physiological abnormality that prevents or slows weight loss (e.g., hypothyroidism, insulin resistance, etc.) (Frank, 2014). It is worth mentioning that clinicians should not assume that individuals with atypical AN are healthier than those with typical AN.

Problems with Atypical AN

Not only is the phenomenon of atypical AN often unnoticed in families, schools, and healthcare settings, it is sadly common for these patients to be praised for their weight loss. Praise comes in the form of compliments about their body's aesthetic and their "dedication to health." Such praise reinforces the disordered eating behavior, which in turn strengthens the cognitions about self-worth and body image and fears about weight gain. Despite the display of reinforcement, organ function continues to erode concurrently over time. Peebles and colleagues (2010) examined the relationship between DSM-IV-TR criteria for EDs, diagnosis, and medical complications. Despite being within a "normal" weight range, results showed that these participants tended to be more medically compromised (requiring hospitalization) than some of their peers who were underweight and diagnosed with AN. They also displayed high rates of complications (18%) once admitted to hospital.

Medical Sequelae of Being Underweight and/or Malnourished

A primary concern when working with individuals who are substantially underweight and/or malnourished is their physical safety and risk of medical complications, which is quite common in many cases of restrictive disorders (i.e., AN, atypical AN, ARFID). Chronic malnutrition and starvation seen in AN (and likely all restrictive disorders) affects virtually every major organ system, and may result in permanent damage or death when not addressed in a timely manner. This is particularly relevant in the case of atypical AN given the prior point that they are often overlooked (Mehler & Brown, 2015; Peebles et al., 2010). Issues of hypotension, bradycardia, and hypothermia often present as the disorder persists (Bulik et al., 2021; Miller et al., 2005), and they pose a serious threat to safety. In addition to the complications linked to a risk of death, the sequelae of chronic low weight impacts dermatological health (Strumia et al., 2005), gastrointestinal functioning (Kamal et al., 1991), the endocrine system (Dalle Grave et al., 2008; Lo Sauro et al., 2008), hematologic functioning (Hütter et al., 2009), neurologic development (Ehrlich et al., 2008), and pulmonary functioning (Gardini-Gardenghi et al., 2009).

The effects that poorer physiological functioning have on growth, bone density, metabolism, and fertility add to the urgency of achieving weight gain goals (Bulik et al., 2021; Fairburn, 2008). Urgency to restore weight is of particular relevance when working with children and adolescents because of the impact of stunted development on their long-term health (Fairburn, 2008; Peebles & Sieke, 2019). However, such concerns could be applicable in all cases of disordered eating that result in extreme malnutrition, regardless of weight. For example, a patient presenting with ARFID and a BMI of 34 whose diet consists of only white flour, fats, and some fruits runs the risk of life-threatening anemia (i.e., requiring a blood transfusion) due to a significant deficiency of iron.

AN is associated with a notable death rate of roughly 5% (Van Eeden et al., 2021), and has been identified as having the second highest mortality rate of all psychiatric illnesses, after opiate use disorder. Individuals with AN have a 9.9-fold increased risk of mortality compared to the general population (Smink et al., 2012). The primary causes of death in patients with AN are suicide and varied medical complications from low body weight and malnutrition (Papadopoulos et al., 2009; Van Eeden et al., 2021). Despite lower mortality rates in recent decades for younger patients, recurrent relapse and psychiatric comorbidity worsened outcomes (Papadopoulos et al., 2009). Put simply, even though we are seeing an improvement in mortality rates, treatment outcomes are still generally undesirable due to recurrent relapse and psychiatric comorbidity.

Given the broad impact of malnutrition, many factors are considered in evaluating physical safety. A review by Miller et al. (2005) showed high rates of complications in AN patients treated in an outpatient setting, informing current recommendations for careful monitoring with regular physical exams and lab assessments by a medical provider to increase safety and reduce risks of complications.

Psychological Sequelae of Low Weight and/or Malnutrition

Perhaps one of the biggest challenges in working with individuals with restrictive EDs is overcoming their psychological "blind spots," also known as anosognosia (i.e., a person being unable to understand and perceive their illness), that present because of malnutrition and low body weight. Many patients are completely unaware of the ways their low weight impacts their executive functioning, interests, emotion regulation, anxiety, perception, obsessionality, preoccupation with food and body image, and mood. The brain requires a lot of energy to function optimally. When individuals are at a low weight and/or malnourished, it becomes difficult for the brain to shift quickly and fluidly between topics (Wang et al., 2021). Concentration and mood are also often impaired in ways that are not always obvious to the underweight person. Specifically, mood is generally low and prone to increased irritability. As a result, thinking is often inflexible and decision-making becomes difficult (Huang & Foldi, 2022) as a sense of anxiety and perseveration is elicited even in relation to relatively small details (Fairburn, 2008; Wang et al., 2021; Wilsdon & Wade, 2006). There is a notable paradox to the idea that many individuals engage in undereating as a means of emotion regulation and distress tolerance. However, this coping skill further inhibits their ability to emotionally regulate and tolerate distress. The relationship between undereating, emotion regulation, and distress tolerance will be elaborated further in Chapter 10.

Similarly, one of the most notable psychological changes in patients who are significantly underweight is an increase in obsessionality (Godier & Park, 2014). This effect often presents as an impairing level of rigidity and inflexibility regarding routines, cleanliness, and orderliness (Casper, 1990; Raney et al., 2008; Shafran, 2002; Wonderlich et al., 2005). Compulsive or ritualized eating behaviors typically emerge as well (e.g., eating slowly, chewing a certain number of times, eating food in a specific order, etc.). This can become more challenging when the patient already has comorbid OCD. Social functioning, an element essential to the psychological well-being of humans, suffers greatly when people are significantly underweight (Fairburn, 2008). Patients gradually become increasingly self-focused and eventually socially withdraw. Increased social isolation is associated with general psychological deterioration (Robb et al., 2020), in addition to the high suicide rate found in patients with AN (Papadopoulos et al., 2009; Van Eeden et al., 2021).

Dietary Needs

Underweight/malnourished individuals have varying dietary needs based on laboratory results, which determine potential complications from nutritional deficiencies or organ malfunction. Thorough assessment and reassessment is necessary during treatment, and dietary needs may take priority over psychological interventions if medical safety is at risk. Additionally, higher calorie diets increase the rate of weight gain and shorten hospital stays (Garber et al., 2013). Restored weight is especially preferred in adolescent cases because of the already malleable state of their physiology at that age. Additionally, many individuals with restrictive EDs (AN in particular) become hypermetabolic during weight restoration (Baracos, 2001; Walker et al., 1979), which requires a high calorie diet to maintain the desired healthy weight (Weltzin et al., 1991).

While prioritizing dietary needs for underweight/malnourished individuals is necessary for medical reasons, it can hinder overall treatment. Firstly, compliance with dietary needs may simply not be feasible. Compliance can be challenging due to factors such as food shortages, financial strain, logistical barriers, and the absence of caretakers. Noncompliance can increase tension during mealtimes and impact ED recovery. It is not surprising that individuals with co-occurring EDs and OCD will have obsessive thoughts and rigidity about the food they consume (Frank et al; 2012; Sternheim et al., 2011). This obsessionality may present as a hyperfixation or set of rules about calories, macronutrients, food quality (i.e., organic or "clean" versus processed), times of eating, avoidance of food groups or eating scenarios, etc.

Guidelines for High-Calorie Diets

It is well documented that effective treatment for AN is primarily defined by remission of low body weight and starvation efforts in addition to improved sense of body image. Most cases require the patient to gain a significant amount of weight that varies in range based on the severity at the time of treatment and one's premorbid weight (e.g., 10–40 lbs in most cases). As one would imagine, the more weight needed to achieve remission of symptoms, the more challenging the presentation. Such cases usually require longer treatment, sometimes higher levels of care, and, most notably, high calorie diets (Fairburn, 2008; Weltzin et al., 1991).

There is no set calorie number or range that will work for every person at every stage of their treatment. In fact, it is typical that the calories needed to achieve and maintain goals change throughout treatment (Marzola et al., 2013; Walker et al., 1979). Much of the calorie requirement issue relates to the biology of starvation and metabolism, which is beyond the focus of this book. However, to understand this idea broadly, we must understand the notion that the human body is in a constant fight for homeostasis (Pinel et al., 2000). Our bodies adjust to the environment and conditions in which it finds itself. Perpetual hunger and starvation is trauma to the whole body. The body does not know why it is being deprived of food; it reacts to starvation trauma by changing its daily operations, just as it would in response to being stranded on a desert island, without understanding the cause of the food deprivation. Metabolism slows and fat is stored due to the lack of energy consumed (Woods & Ramsay, 2011) in an attempt to maintain homeostasis and to use energy efficiently for survival.

In the very early stages of refeeding, sometimes there is some immediate weight gain after increasing caloric intake. This is not the case for a non-ED individual eating regularly because the body is in a state of homeostasis. Because an individual with AN has such a low baseline of calories, their weight will likely increase briefly in the early stages of refeeding. As more food becomes available and is consumed on a consistent basis, the brain signals that metabolism can increase, potentially stymying weight gain. Medical providers are not clear on exactly why this happens, but the phenomenon of hypermetabolism is almost universal to this phase of weight restoration (Marzola et al., 2013). At this point, the underweight or malnourished person's diet must be adjusted (i.e., calorie increase) to continue to yield the desired weight gain. Achieving this continued caloric intake is complicated in AN and other restrictive ED presentations by three primary variables: (1) gastrointestinal distress and extreme fullness with even a "normal" number of calories let alone the increased amount, (2) one's refusal to consume the prescribed calories needed to achieve desired weight gain, and (3) hypermetabolic states as weight increases. As previously stated, the refeeding process requires increasing calories to continue gaining weight as the body gets closer to the desired healthy weight (Marzola et al., 2013; Walker, 1979). A healthy weight range is usually identified by a combination of variables, such as a return of menstrual cycle (if applicable), pediatric growth charts, immediate family members weight ranges/body types, premorbid weight, medical findings (e.g., metabolic laboratory panel, heart rate, orthostates, etc.), and psychological functioning. Not all such data points are available in all cases, but when they are, clinicians ought to identify a goal weight range based on a compilation of such information.

In early studies of weight gain in AN, researchers found that the caloric needs could range from 4,000 to 9,000 calories per day based on the person's sex, height, and degree to which they were underweight as compared to their healthy range (Keys & Brožek, 1953; Passmore et al., 1955). Similarly, Russell and Mezey (1962) reported that a mean caloric intake of 7,500 per day is needed to achieve weight gain. Further, Walker and colleagues (1979) found that starting weights predicted how many calories one would need to gain weight. Results of more recent studies are consistent with such findings (e.g., Garber et al., 2013). A higher range of calories is often consumed in a medical inpatient hospital stay, and the more typical range for refeeding in an outpatient setting ranges from 3,000 to 5,000 calories per day. APA guidelines do not specify a calorie range for outpatients (Marzola et al., 2013); thus, the 3,000–5,000 range is an anecdotal clinical observation from working with many outpatients who have recently transitioned from an inpatient hospitalization.

Many clinicians and families hope that once weight has been restored and metabolism has returned to usual functioning, the estimated caloric range needed for maintenance is comparable to non-ED peers of the same age and sex (e.g., roughly between 2,000 and 3,000 calories per day, depending on activity level). This may take a long period of time for some, and it may not occur for all patients. Bulik and colleagues (2021) discuss metabolic abnormalities in patients with AN at length as it pertains to genetics, stating that some individuals with AN have metabolism-based genes that make sustained weight maintenance (once restored) quite difficult even in the absence of restriction. Thus, they make the case to classify AN as a metabo-psychiatric disorder.

Food Density and Diet Variety

Another interesting finding related to weight gain, dietary needs, and positive outcomes in AN patients relates to food density and diet variety. Schebendach and colleagues (2008) examined weight-restored women with AN and found that lower food density and diet variety was associated with weight loss and relapse once monitoring of food intake stopped. Most notably, the number of calories consumed was not associated with poorer outcomes. Their findings showed a significant difference in fat consumption between the treatment success group and the treatment failure group. It is common for those with AN to avoid high-density foods (e.g., French fries, milkshakes) in their diets and to prefer to consume large quantities of low-density foods (i.e., vegetables, lean meats, etc.) to achieve their calorie requirement for weight gain. The reason for this preference is usually a combination of how the foods feel physiologically in the body, a persistent fear of weight gain (despite being the agreed upon goal), beliefs related to indulgence or gluttony that get triggered when eating food that tastes good and cause a release of dopamine in the brain, and general societal messaging about "good" vs. "bad" foods. This approach of consuming low-density foods can be effective when calorie intake is monitored closely, but it can be challenging to maintain over the long term as monitoring decreases. Patients may lose motivation to eat large portions of low-density foods, and this avoidance of high-density foods can negatively impact treatment outcomes and long-term prognosis. Gradual weight loss may occur over time as the patient reduces their intake of low-density foods and continues to avoid high-density foods. ED specialists are all too aware of this common challenge.

Given the common occurrence of denial for the serious nature of the problem and the distorted view of food and weight, it is clear why many patients struggle to comply with high-calorie diets without closely calculated and monitored accountability by providers and supports. Diet noncompliance poses a challenge in treatment, which is only exacerbated by a comorbid OCD diagnosis wherein corresponding exposure-based interventions are indicated. When we combine what we know about diet noncompliance with Bulik et al.'s (2021) work about the genetics involved in metabolism and AN, it makes sense that clinicians encourage significant weight gain early in treatment with the goal weight being at the higher end of the person's range. In other words, when we have patients who are already working with a faster metabolism, making weight gain and maintenance harder, it seems wise to want to have "cushion calories" and "cushion weight" to account for the inevitable burning and loss that is likely to occur.

High caloric intake not only leads to quicker remission of symptoms, it can also aid in producing higher weights, which indirectly acts as a relapse prevention intervention.

As noted earlier, Garber et al. (2013) found that higher calorie diets led to both quicker weight gain and shorter hospital stays in adolescents. Fast weight gain is particularly relevant for providers to consider given that the best prognosis for AN occurs when there is a short duration between treatment initiation and weight gain as well as for the duration of illness overall. Lock and Le Grange (2001) recommend 2.4 kg (5 lbs) within the first month of treatment for the best prognosis. Additionally, shorter hospital stays are more cost efficient and preferred for optimal adolescent development. Although early weight gain is critical, it must be achieved with careful consideration. In fact, Garber et al.'s (2013) study described a potential problem documented in the treatment of AN: the refeeding syndrome.

Refeeding Syndrome

Research has documented refeeding syndrome as a life-threatening risk within treatment for AN (Skowrońska et al., 2019). During World War II, individuals experiencing starvation had low blood pressure and reduced heart muscle (Machado et al., 2009). These effects are particularly problematic when refeeding occurs too quickly – cardiovascular collapse can occur because it is difficult for the smaller heart muscle to effectively manage the increase in blood volume that happens as one undergoes a significant (and rapid) increase of caloric intake as seen in AN treatment (Hearing, 2004; Machado et al., 2009; Skowrońska et al., 2019). To ensure the stability and effective functioning of the cardiovascular system as caloric intake increases, the body needs close medical monitoring within the first few weeks of refeeding.

The risk of encountering refeeding syndrome has led many clinicians to err on the conservative side by prescribing lower calorie diets at the start of treatment. However, numerous studies (e.g., Doyle et al., 2010, Hartmann et al., 2007; Le Grange et al., 2014; Lock et al., 2006; Madden et al., 2015), as mentioned in Chapter 6, indicated that early weight gain (from high calorie diets) and/or regulated eating are associated with optimal recovery outcomes in addition to an immediate reduction in psychiatric symptoms (Wilson et al., 2002). Further, Garber et al. (2013) did not find any cases of refeeding syndrome with their prescribed high-calorie diets in a study on hospitalized adolescents. They utilized a phosphate supplement as a proactive intervention to mitigate onset of the refeeding syndrome. Consequently, these results support aggressive refeeding in AN treatment, especially in hospital settings.

Outpatient settings present higher risk of refeeding syndrome and greater challenges for providers, including clinician anxiety due to the significant health consequences, increased mortality rate, and liability of treating this population. To reduce clinician anxiety, outpatient providers can have patients seen by a medical provider regularly (i.e., once or twice a week) until sufficient weight gain is achieved. Logistics regarding the collaboration process with medical providers will be highlighted further in Chapter 8.

Impact of Low Body Weight and Malnourishment on Exposure

As this chapter highlights, attending to low body weights and malnourishment ought to be prioritized in treatment from the start. We would go as far to say that the only other target areas that may take precedence are active suicidal ideation and abuse. Does this mean providers ought to hold off on conducting exposures and instead solely work on dietary restriction when patients are underweight and/or malnourished? Not necessarily. While it is safe to assume that the neurocognitive state of a person who is currently underweight and/or malnourished may hinder the effects of exposure-based interventions, there is no evidence to halt exposures completely. That said, there are a few points to consider.

Considerations for Exposure Therapy

The effects of starvation and anosognosia in restrictive EDs make exposure therapy a challenging task for clinicians, given the high anxiety and low motivation presentation (Fairburn, 2008). Although the science does indicate that underweight and/or malnourished patients can benefit from exposure, we argue that because exposure works best when it is volitional, it may not be a desirable option for malnourished or underweight patients, who may engage in mental rituals that undermine its effects (Farrell et al., 2019). The baseline anxiety of such patients is already higher than average, leading to slower or less robust habituation and inhibitory learning at the start of treatment. The focus of exposures should be primarily geared toward increased food intake and weight gain until sufficient weight is restored and the brain and body are on their way to optimal functioning. Exposures for co-occurring OCD should be deferred until later in treatment.

In Summary

It is important for clinicians to consider the specific factors and challenges highlighted throughout this chapter that are involved in treatment when patients present as under-weight and/or malnourished. Both underweight and malnutrition can be caused by psycho-logical factors, such as restrictive EDs (AN, ARFID, and ON) or chronic anxiety, and can have significant implications for treatment and overall health. Prolonged periods of malnu-trition can lead to weight loss and negative impacts on brain and organ function. Treatment for underweight and malnutrition often involves addressing dietary concerns and incorp-orating medical care into the treatment plan, and may also involve addressing co-occurring conditions such as EDs and OCD. The rationale for behavioral interventions that yield weight gain and increased food volume and variety in patients' diets has been made clear throughout this chapter. Because the reason for patients being malnourished and/or underweight is rooted in fears and aversions to food and weight-related variables, exposure therapy presents as a suitable match for treatment.

Chapter

8

Provider Collaboration in Eating Disorder Treatment

The two primary empirically supported treatments for EDs – CBT-E and FBT – suggest having a limited treatment team consisting of a primary therapist focusing on changing eating habits along with weight and body image issues, a medical professional to monitor stability, and a psychiatrist for managing any accompanying diagnoses through medication (if necessary). Dietitians typically should be used as consultants to the primary therapist on an as-needed basis, and other types of therapy should be suspended during CBT-E and FBT. Treatment providers can be compared to skilled chefs who believe that a meal will turn out better when there are not "too many cooks in the kitchen." This approach aims to reduce the risk of conflicting messages among providers and treatment fatigue for patients. While this approach has been used in most clinical trials of CBT-E and FBT, it has not yet become standard practice in ED treatment. Despite evidence supporting the efficacy of CBT-E and FBT, outdated ideas about ED maintenance and treatment persist in the healthcare community, thereby creating treatment challenges, especially when the patient also has a co-occurring diagnosis of OCD.

Barriers within the Multidisciplinary Treatment Team Approach

Despite evidence for a limited treatment team approach, many providers hold the belief that "more is better" regarding ED treatment services. This belief is particularly relevant in countries with private (and less regulated) healthcare systems, such as in the United States. The idea of ED patients having a comprehensive team is widely accepted as ideal treatment conditions among many ED providers and patients alike. This team typically consists of a primary therapist, a medical provider, a psychiatrist, a dietitian, and, in some cases, an additional family therapist or experiential therapist (i.e., art or dance/movement therapist). Some programming also include peer mentors and family peer supports with lived experience of an ED. This treatment infrastructure is employed by many ED treatment centers across the United States despite being absent from the leading treatments.

Conflicting Ideas

Multidisciplinary teams may result in the "too many cooks" in the kitchen problem. When there are too many cooks, each with different training, conflicting ideas about what the desired meal may be, which ingredients are needed for the best taste, and what techniques will be most time-efficient can arise. In treatment, members of the same treatment team may disagree about weight goals, how to achieve said weight goals, whether exposures should include collaborative weighing, if and when there should be a focus on self-esteem and body image, and how long the patient should be in treatment.

There are many vital questions that need to be asked in ED treatment, and the answers can become "blurry" when there are many providers on the treatment team. In summary, more "cooks in the kitchen" means more opinions (that may conflict), more appointments, increasing burnout risk, and data that could become lost in translation. Additionally, OCD treatment is niche-specific, requiring thorough understanding of what interventions are needed to remit symptoms and what interventions or strategies serve as maintenance and exacerbating variables. Thus, when an individual has co-occurring OCD, it is likely that they will employ checking behaviors and other forms of reassurance seeking throughout the treatment process. Untrained yet well-intentioned providers (i.e., dietitians) or peer mentors, for example, may very well feed right into this maintenance cycle by offering otherwise helpful advice, education, or answers to questions.

Communication and Logistic Barriers

As Chapter 7 briefly mentioned, cases of significant medical complications because of low body weight and/or malnutrition are best managed with more collateral contact between the primary therapist and the medical provider. However, difficulties in coordinating consistent and ongoing collaboration between multiple treatment providers can be problematic for ED patients and their support network. Heightened emotional distress, malnutrition and low body weight (Fairburn, 2008; Wilsdon & Wade, 2006), and lack of motivation can contribute to misinterpretation and loss of information, leading to mixed messages and misunderstandings both between patients and providers and among the providers. The need for accurate and clear communication between all members of the treatment team is crucial to ensure effective treatment.

The Gap between ED Research and Practice in Healthcare

Despite the growing empirical data supporting CBT-E and FBT's efficacy in producing positive treatment outcomes, antiquated ideas about ED maintenance and treatment persist in the health care community. This is elaborated further in Chapter 11.

Assessment of Severity

Regardless of studies (e.g., Peebles et al., 2010) that have debunked the oversimplified association between pathology severity and body weight, providers still tend to sound the loudest alarms about severity when patients are underweight and malnourished. This may be due to media representation of EDs, societal stigma, weight bias, and the well-known medical risks and complications associated with these disorders that were mentioned in Chapter 7. Generalist providers may be more likely than ED specialists to believe that more treatment is better for ED patients. These generalists, who may not be familiar with the latest research on ED treatment, may also make recommendations that are not necessarily indicated in the literature, such as referring patients to a dietitian or encouraging higher levels of care when not typically indicated.

Utilization of Dietitians

Despite clear evidence that addressing current problematic eating and weight behaviors is key to achieving remission of EDs (CBT-E and FBT), the belief that EDs stem from underlying psychological issues persists in healthcare and popular culture. This perpetuates stigma and reinforces the outdated idea that psychotherapy for EDs should focus on underlying causes rather than eating and weight-related behaviors. As a result, many healthcare providers in the United States often refer ED patients to dietitians for nutritional counseling first, before consultation with a mental health specialist in EDs. This may be due to this referral carrying less stigma than mental health. Outpatient treatment from a mental health expert in EDs is often seen as a secondary or tertiary option. Even when referrals to both a dietitian and a mental health provider are made, the dietitian is often primarily responsible for monitoring weight, providing food and weight education, and developing a plan to improve eating and weight behaviors. Some ED therapists may also delegate eating and weight behaviors to dietitians, or not prioritize this based on personal preference or theoretical orientation.

This practice has several negative implications for treatment outcomes and healthcare costs. Dietitians may lack specific training in exposure therapy, making it difficult for them to effectively address disordered eating behaviors and beliefs. Patients may become stuck in a cycle of negative thoughts and behaviors related to eating and weight. While dietitians do have expertise in food science and nutrition, they may not be equipped to address the complex behavioral and cognitive mechanisms that maintain disordered eating. Additionally, this approach can be especially problematic for patients with co-occurring OCD, as nutrition programs typically do not include training on OCD. A lack of training could result in a dietitian not recognizing when their interventions may be worsening the symptoms of OCD. For example, educating a person with OCD about the importance of fats and carbohydrates in their diet may provide temporary relief, but may also reinforce the OCD, preventing the person from tolerating uncertainty. This could result in a strengthening of the illness overall, creating further problems in treatment and in the person's life outside of treatment. Dietitians who lack training in behavioral learning principles may negatively impact ED patients by encouraging avoidance of monitoring food and weight (using "blight weights," or stepping on the scale backwards at appointments). This approach may provide comfort in the moment but prevent corrective and inhibitory learning, limit accurate meal planning, and hinder the return of hunger cues, all of which are critical for recovery.

In Summary

Both of the two primary empirically supported treatments for EDs (CBT-E and FBT) recommend that the treatment team be limited to a few key members, including a primary therapist who focuses on changing eating behaviors, weight, and related body image concerns, a medical provider to monitor stability, and a psychiatrist for medication-based management of any comorbid diagnoses (if applicable). Dietitians may be used as consultants to the primary therapist on an as-needed basis, but other types of therapy should be suspended during CBT-E and FBT. This limited team approach is intended to reduce the risk of conflicting messages among providers, miscommunication, reinforcing of safety behaviors or other maintaining variables, and treatment fatigue for patients. While this approach has been used in most clinical trials of CBT-E and FBT, it is not yet standard practice in ED treatment. Despite evidence supporting the efficacy of CBT-E and FBT, outdated ideas about ED maintenance and treatment persist in the healthcare community, which can be a challenge in treatment, especially when the patient also has a co-occurring diagnosis of OCD.

Chapter 9

Impact of Eating Disorder Treatment on Obsessive-Compulsive Symptoms

This chapter highlights components of the most commonly used empirically supported ED treatments (i.e., CBT-E and FBT) that may not be suitable or may need adaptations for patients who also have OCD. These points will be based on observations from clinical practice. Primary aspects of evidence-based ED treatments discussed in this chapter relate to parental control in FBT, collaborative weighing, self-monitoring and eating schedules/meal plans, and psychoeducation about food and weight.

Parental Control

In our clinical experience, clinicians have identified patterns among patients and parents who have not successfully responded to FBT interventions, with the most commonly reported barrier being an increase in OCD symptoms (i.e., "it made the OCD worse"). The underlying mechanisms of FBT that aggravate OCD symptoms remain largely unknown; however, through clinical observations, patients have reported that "the preoccupation with numbers and exactness worsened towards food and became about things other than food." Most notably from our clinical observation, obsessionality expanded to concerns about exercise/movement and other topics within the morality domain of OCD.

Case Example: Margot

Margot is a 17-year-old female who presented with OCD and AN. She had undergone FBT (unsuccessfully) and subsequently became increasingly obsessive about productivity and feeling as though she ought to suffer, equating this with being a good, moral person. Any occurrence of relaxation, making her life easier, pleasure, or enjoyment was met with much difficulty and heightened emotional distress, as these equated to indulgence and laziness. Similarly, she believed that exercising her privilege in life meant that she was "indulgent" and thus a bad person.

As a result, Margot engaged in the following behaviors: (1) stand whenever possible; (2) eat as blandly as possible; (3) drink only liquids throughout the day unless forced (in an attempt to save solid foods for night time when she believed that she had "earned" more enjoyable energy consumption); (4) wear old, ripped clothes instead of the new clothes her parents bought her; (5) fill every moment of her free time with either movement, charity-based work, or schoolwork; and (6) purposefully put extra heavy textbooks in her backpack at school to compensate for sitting down throughout the day in her classes. Margot had difficulty seeing the lack of connection between engaging in these behaviors and what it means to be a good person. Margot continually failed to comply with treatment recommendations even though treatment noncompliance meant that her mother's money for treatment was essentially going to "waste," a paradox often seen in OCD. Margot also encountered many problems with the use of the scale in treatment, in addition to the many "unknowns" in treatment such as content within food and whether or not she was ever eating "more than needed."

According to Margot's OCD's logic, this noncompliance should have activated her intrusive thoughts. In fact, she expressed an awareness of this "wastefulness" and guilt about the fact that those less privileged than her do not even have the opportunity to see a psychologist, let alone receive specialized treatment in the areas of concern. However, this acknowledgment and guilt did not yield behavior change, indicating the level of rigidity often seen in overlapping OCD and ED presentations.

We have some thoughts about why cases like Margot's exist. Clinicians and researchers have identified that a need for perfectionism, overestimating the level of threat, having difficulty tolerating uncertainty, and a desire to control one's intrusive thoughts play a role in the maintenance of OCD (Hezel & McNally, 2016; Hezel & Simpson, 2019) As such, ED treatment interventions that result in greater uncertainty and less control may contribute to exacerbated OCD symptoms, at least in the short term. We must state here that there is not an empirical basis for this hypothesis, but rather a notable clinical observation.

As stated in Chapter 2, the theoretical basis of FBT for adolescents with AN involves the assumption that adolescents with AN are unable to feed themselves properly due to starvation and low body weight. As a result, parents are given control over the adolescent's food and exercise in order to achieve weight gain quickly. However, the lack of control and increased uncertainty experienced by adolescents during FBT may be related to increased OCD symptoms and poor treatment outcomes for those with comorbid OCD. The level of fear and preoccupation may be greater for these individuals due to their heightened baseline level of obsessionality, anxiety sensitivity, and distress tolerance. While there is no data to support this notion, it is possible that the needs of these individuals may be better met with some modifications to traditional FBT or with CBT-E, where the patient voluntarily chooses to make behavioral changes.

Collaborative Weighing

Another notable intervention that is central to both CBT-E and FBT is collaborative weighing. Although neither treatment describes the use of collaborative weighing as exposure therapy, it may function like an exposure intervention, as described in Chapter 6. In-session collaborative weighing can look similar to the ritual prevention and exposure elements found in effective OCD treatment. For weighing in FBT, the therapist may want to weigh the patient alone to form some alliance; however, despite this attempt at collaboration, an adolescent with AN likely does not want to engage in treatment, or maybe even be weighed, therefore making it an involuntary exposure intervention that is less likely to be successful. Thus, it has the potential for greater anxiety, uncertainty, and frustration, and less efficacy as an exposure intervention.

As discussed in Chapter 2 and further elaborated on in Section III of this book, both FBT and CBT-E use collaborative weighing as a tool to track progress and monitor weight gain. However, the goals of and approach to this intervention differ between the two treatments. CBT-E uses collaborative weighing to reduce the emotional significance of weight and shape, teaching individuals distress tolerance and a more neutral relationship with the scale. In contrast, FBT-AN uses collaborative weighing solely as a monitor for progress, with emotions and cognitions related to weight and the scale not directly addressed. Tracking weight and eating in FBT and CBT-E may be problematic for ED patients with comorbid OCD. They may fixate on numbers even in the case of minor changes, and the chart tracking may become a new obsessional domain or a means of reassurance, rather than exposure therapy. In the case of Margot, her fixation with numbers related to her weight ended up branching out to other domains. Similarly, collaborative weighing served as reassurance rather than exposure when she underwent CBT-E as a young adult. This highlights the need for caution and an individualized treatment approach in cases with comorbid OCD. The same can be said for the manner in which planning and monitoring of eating occurs.

Self-Monitoring, Eating Schedules, and Meal Plans

Though neither treatment manual uses the term "meal plan," both CBT-E and FBT discuss meal planning and eating schedules. Both models view the continuation of these behaviors as a key factor in maintaining the illness. Self-monitoring helps therapists identify ways to intervene in eating behaviors, and the implementation of meal plans with eating schedules are crucial in attacking maladaptive eating behaviors from the start of treatment.

In CBT-E, patients track their eating behavior using a log provided by the therapist. The log includes information on day, date, time, food, and location, and related thoughts, feelings, and triggers. Patients are encouraged to fill out the log as soon after eating as possible, with a focus on the context and experience of eating (versus specific foods, calorie counting, weighing food, or portion sizes). FBT for AN may involve a dietitian consultation for setting caloric intake goals and coaching parents on recommended foods to meet refeeding goals. The goal is to promote weight gain and empower parents to feed their child enough. Calories are adjusted as weight changes, with no daily monitoring logs.

Similar to the problem of collaborative weighing, the use of self-monitoring in treating adolescents with comorbid OCD and EDs may pose a threat due to the rigidity surrounding numbers and meal times. This can exacerbate OCD symptoms and lead to compulsive behaviors. The self-monitoring record may also serve as a source of reassurance for the individual, triggering increased obsessions and distrust. Some of these problems came up in the case of Margot. The treatment team must take the individual's OCD symptoms into account and work with the patient and their family to address potential triggers and challenges.

Psychoeducation about Food and Weight

Psychoeducation about food and weight is a key component of Stage 1 in CBT-E, which aims to address faulty beliefs and assumptions that individuals with EDs may have developed about the relationship between food consumption and weight changes. In contrast, FBT education about the effects of being underweight and malnourished and the safety and long-term implications of the ED is directed more toward the parents than the patient. However, the adolescent may be present unwillingly, making these education messages noncollaborative, which may lead to anxiety and distress throughout the first phase of FBT. Furthermore, the adolescent may not realize the beneficial implications of weight gain, for example, given that they are likely still engaging in rituals and safety behaviors.

Psychoeducation about food and weight is a crucial part of Stage 1 in CBT-E and FBT, but it may lead to anxiety and distress in the adolescent, particularly in the case of comorbid OCD. In CBT-E, psychoeducation addresses faulty beliefs and assumptions, while in FBT it educates parents about the effects of being underweight and malnourished. This psychoeducation has been shown to be impactful in BN and BED with regard to behavior change (as illustrated in Chapter 6) and neutral to helpful in AN and ARFID. However, the psychoeducation in ERP for comorbid OCD is limited to avoid serving as reassurance. Instead, the focus is on the relationship between obsessions and compulsions and the need for exposure therapy. ERP therapists tend to say something along the lines of "I'm going to tell you X once [usually some type of psychoeducation], but I am not going to say this again in the interest of not reassuring your OCD." The impact of psychoeducation on behavior change in individuals with non-OCD EDs is positive, but in those with comorbid OCD it is argued to be damaging. The consequences of psychoeducation may be less relevant in FBT with co-occurring OCD as the information is directed to the parents, and the adolescent may be less likely to absorb and use it as reassurance.

In Summary

This chapter aimed to highlight some of the most important features of empirically supported ED treatments that may pose a problem for patients with co-occurring OCD. The implication here is not to assume that such interventions ought to be forfeited altogether, but rather that they should be modified in some ways. In cases where modification may not be warranted, clinicians should at the very least be mindful of how the person's OCD may progress and continue to assess symptoms throughout treatment, even if OCD is not being directly treated at that time.

10 The Relationship between Eating, Distress Tolerance, and Emotion Regulation in Obsessive-Compulsive Disorder

People with OCD often engage in behaviors that help them avoid or escape anxious or distressed feelings. These behaviors can include typical compulsions seen in OCD (i.e., handwashing, checking), as well as other maladaptive behaviors such as substance use or problematic eating (i.e., bingeing, frequent emotional eating). These eating patterns can be a form of experiential avoidance, or the attempt to change or avoid negative thoughts, emotions, or physical sensations, even if it causes harm. Individuals with OCD may also have high levels of anxiety sensitivity (AS), intolerance of uncertainty (IU), perfectionism, and low distress tolerance (DT), which can be maintained by avoidance behaviors. These behaviors can hinder building tolerance of these factors and exacerbate their negative effects. This chapter will explore the relationship between DT and related constructs, OCD, and problematic eating patterns.

What Is DT?

DT (previously discussed in Chapter 3) refers to a person's ability to cope with negative emotions. It includes one's perception of their own ability to handle negative emotions, the intensity of the negative emotions they experience, and their desire to change their emotional state when distressed (Simons & Gaher, 2005). Low DT, also known as distress intolerance, is a limited capacity for enduring negative emotional experiences and a tendency to become overly reactive to stress and distress. This vulnerability is often associated with borderline personality disorder (BPD), where a combination of biological predisposition, an emotionally invalidating childhood, and a tendency to use avoidance coping strategies leads to a low capacity for tolerating distress (Linehan, 1993). Low DT has been linked to a range of dysregulated behaviors and psychological disorders, including self-injury, substance use, gambling, BN, BPD, antisocial disorder, and anxiety disorders (Anestis et al., 2007, Buckner et al., 2007, Daughters et al., 2005, Daughters et al., 2008, Gratz et al., 2006, Michel et al., 2016; Nock & and Mendes, 2008; Peterson et al., 2014).

In the literature, DT is described as a higher-order factor of affect intolerance and sensitivities (see Bernstein et al., 2009 for review) and is thought to have various lower-order constructs, including emotional dysregulation, IU, AS, negative urgency (NU), and experiential avoidance (EA) (Conway et al., 2021; Simons & Gaher, 2005). The relationship between these constructs is not well understood, but some researchers speculate that they may be distinct (Leyro et al., 2010; Zvolensky et al., 2010) and have a synergistic effect on emotions and behaviors within disorders (Van Eck et al., 2017). Brief explanations of these related lower-order constructs are described here for a more comprehensive understanding of DT.

Lower-Order Constructs

Emotional regulation (ER), EA, UI, AS, and NU are constructs related to distress intolerance, as they all involve an inability to cope with negative emotions or experiences. ER refers to managing and controlling emotions to have an adaptive response (Gross & Thompson, 2007). Poor ER skills can result in emotional dysregulation and a belief of being incapable of handling negative triggers, leading to maladaptive coping strategies and a reduction in DT (Gross, 2002; Naragon-Gainey et al., 2017). People with poor ER skills are more likely to experience frequent episodes of emotional dysregulation (Van Eck et al., 2017). EA is the avoidance of internal experiences (i.e., thoughts, emotions, and somatic sensations) through escape behaviors (e.g., constant use of one's phone as a distraction) (Hayes et al., 1996), and IU refers to difficulty coping with unpredictability and change (Obsessive Compulsive Cognitions Working Group, 1997 in Clark, 2020). IU often involves a negative mood state and repetitive negative thoughts about undesirable outcomes. AS is susceptibility to negative affect and fear of the consequences of anxiety. Further, AS is characterized by an excessive concern about the potentially catastrophic consequences of experiencing anxiety (Reiss et al., 1986). NU refers to acting impulsively when upset (Racine et al., 2017) and is similar to low DT. Not only do people believe they cannot handle their negative feelings, they also have the urge to fix or avoid these feelings as quickly as possible.

DT and OCD

Low DT is significantly associated with various anxiety disorders, including GAD, social anxiety, EDs, and obsessive-compulsive symptoms (Anestis et al., 2007; Keough et al., 2010; Norr et al., 2013; Zvolensky et al., 2010). Research has indicated that low DT may play a role in the development and maintenance of obsessions in individuals with OCD (Macatee et al., 2013). Studies have found that DT is a distinct predictor of OCD symptoms, even after accounting for anxiety symptoms, depressive symptoms, and AS (Cougle et al., 2011; Keough et al., 2010). In addition, low DT has been found to be significantly correlated with obsessions, and has been shown to predict the frequency of obsessions in nonclinical samples (Cougle et al., 2012, 2011). The related construct of NU has also been shown to be highly correlated with obsessing symptoms and thought control in a study by Gay et al. (2011). Additionally, there is evidence indicating that the fear of negative emotions and AS are strongly related to OCD symptoms (Deacon & Abramowitz, 2006; McCubbin & Sampson, 2006).

As mentioned in Chapter 3, negative appraisals and dysfunctional beliefs about intrusive thoughts are key factors in the development and maintenance of obsessive thinking in individuals with OCD (Rachman, 1997). These individuals often misinterpret their intrusive thoughts as negative (e.g., bad, scary, or dangerous) and discount how common such thoughts are in the general population (Rachman, 1997). They may also have negative appraisals of themselves based on the content of their thoughts (e.g., "I am a bad person"; "I may hurt someone"). Such beliefs about their inability to withstand the distress associated with the intrusive thought may intensify the individual's impulse to engage in maladaptive strategies or compulsions (i.e., safety/escape behaviors), which will ultimately maintain the intrusive thoughts and contribute to the development of obsessions.

Eating for DT and ER

In addition to typical behaviors associated with anxiety (e.g., avoidance, compulsions), people may also manage distress and anxiety by eating or avoiding food (e.g., restricting, bingeing, emotional eating) to regulate their emotions. There is significant empirical support for the association between intense emotional states and eating behavior in both BN and BED (i.e., bingeing; Agras & Telch, 1998), as well as for AN (i.e., dietary restriction; Brockmeyer et al., 2012). Less is known about ARFID as it relates to DT and ER specifically; however, Zucker et al. (2019) found an association between issues of self-regulation and children with ARFID. This link between negative emotional states and eating behaviors may be supported by research on alexithymia (difficulty identifying and expressing feelings or emotions) with EDs (Christie et al., 2000; Cochrane et al., 1993). The presence of alexithymia in ED patients may suggest that overeating or undereating can be used as a maladaptive strategy to avoid feelings in those with low DT and stress management deficits.

BN and BED

Overeating as a coping mechanism has been documented in patients with BN and BED (Agras & Telch, 1998; Waters et al., 2000). Negative emotional states increase loss of food control in women with BED (Agras & Telch, 1998) and predict binges in patients with BN (Waters et al., 2000). Low DT (perceived inability to tolerate negative emotions) explains a significant portion of dysregulated eating behaviors in BN (Anestis et al., 2007). The case of "Hanna" illustrates this relationship.

Hanna

Hanna is a 19-year-old college student who presented to treatment for BED that had developed within the past year. She had a higher weight as a child and her family members would remind her of this. As a result, she always tried to eat less, but then would end up eating certain foods (i.e., "junk" foods) in secret to avoid comments from family. Food gradually became a source of emotional comfort and her brain formed a connection between emotional dysregulation (including boredom) and eating junk foods. Upon assessing the timeline, she stated that bingeing had become a way of obtaining relief from other areas of her life that had been causing notable distress. Upon further inquiry, it became clear that she had very impairing OCD. She became instantly tearful when discussing some of the intrusive thoughts she had been having about sexuality, pedophilia, and the possibility of one day developing schizophrenia. She engaged in a lot of reassurance seeking compulsions, in addition to avoidance of many stimuli that trigger obsessional content. She had no idea that what she had been experiencing was OCD. She spoke about her binges increasing in frequency as her obsessive thoughts worsened. She stated that this was the only method that had provided at least some short-term relief.

Collaboratively prioritizing disorder treatment is important in cases like these (see Chapter 14 for more on assessment). In the case of Hanna, BED and OCD were treated separately due to limited overlap in content (unlike the case of Margot). To ensure that exposure therapy could be fully experienced, binge-eating was prohibited before/after therapy and homework exposures (to prevent "numbing out"). The rationale was understood and she was successful in implementing exposures without bingeing. Overall, Hanna's OCD was treated with ERP using a combination of imaginal and in vivo exposures and prevention of reassurance (i.e., via internet searching). BED was then treated with CBT-E, but rigid self-monitoring and seeking reassurance from the therapist were challenges. Family reinforcement of weight loss also hindered binge-episode remission.

AN and Restrictive Disorders

Dietary restriction in AN may be linked to DT. Affect intolerance and restriction have fewer studies, but starvation and underweight effects on mood and cognition are well known (Kaye et al., 2004), as stated in Chapter 7. AN patients report that starvation effects (e.g., brain fog, poor concentration) and features such as preoccupation with weight/body/food intake distract from negative thoughts and feelings (Brockmeyer et al., 2012). Perpetual starvation worsens DT and manages ER by creating emotional blunting.

DT and Eating Theories

The first model, known as the blocking model (e.g., Lacey & Moureli, 1986; Reiser, 1990; Root & Fallon, 1989), suggests that people may use behaviors such as bingeing to temporarily block out negative emotions. This model was initially developed to explain binge eating, but has also been applied to AN (Corstorphine, 2006). The "escape from awareness" model (Heatherton & Baumeister, 1991), also known as cognitive narrowing, proposes that bingeing may be a consequence of attempts to escape from self-awareness and negative emotions. Blocking and escape from awareness are two theories that have been proposed to explain the relationship between eating and negative emotions. According to Heatherton and Baumeister (1991), the high standards and criticism that some women face, particularly about their appearance, may motivate them to escape from their awareness in order to avoid the negative feelings that this pressure may cause. Both models link eating behaviors to an inability to tolerate and regulate during distress, with the blocking model suggesting that bingeing is a strategy to escape negative emotions and the escape from awareness model proposing that bingeing is a result of trying to escape from negative emotions.

Treatment Concerns

It is crucial to identify the use of food or overeating as a coping mechanism for people with OCD as this can impede the progress and effectiveness of exposure therapy and ritual prevention. Exposure therapy can be hindered when an individual uses food or overeating as a way to avoid or escape these fears. This can prolong the recovery process and make it harder to break the cycle of OCD. Furthermore, as OCD patients are more prone to develop EDs, it is vital to be aware of any eating patterns related to anxiety. By addressing these underlying issues, individuals with OCD with food and eating can more fully engage in treatment and make progress in overcoming their OCD symptoms.

In Summary

Individuals with OCD often struggle with tolerating distress and frequently experience comorbidity with EDs (Tyagi et al., 2015). Studies have revealed that people with OCD tend to have abnormal eating habits compared to healthy controls (Çelikel et al., 2009). This abnormal eating pattern can be a way to escape or regulate emotions, avoid negative feelings, and, as a result, sustain maintenance variables in the OCD cycle (e.g., avoidance). In some cases, these eating patterns may be an overlooked coping mechanism or maintenance behavior for individuals with OCD who have difficulty tolerating distress and who try to avoid their intrusive thoughts or negative emotions through escape behaviors. Overall, using food as a form of EA can hinder ERP treatment. Additionally, eating as a coping mechanism, paired with the risk that those with OCD are more vulnerable to developing EDs, puts individuals in this subcategory at risk of developing an ED. Thus, properly assessing this behavior can be crucial for robust treatment and the prevention of EDs.

Poorly Executed Exposures

11

Exposure therapy is a type of psychotherapy aimed at helping a person confront their fears or traumatic memories in a controlled and safe environment. It is used to treat phobias, OCD, PTSD, and anxiety disorders, and is based on the idea that facing and confronting triggers manages reactions and reduces negative feelings. Techniques used include imagining, engaging with, and visiting or talking and thinking about the feared situation. The goal is to help the person learn to cope with their fears and reduce negative emotions. Numerous studies (Hofmann & Smits, 2008; Norton & Price, 2007; Olatunji et al, 2010; Rytwinski, 2012) show the efficacy of exposure therapy alone or combined with other interventions for anxiety and fear. Exposure therapy has been manualized into a treatment for OCD (see Chapter 3) and is recognized as a "well-established treatment" and "frontline treatment" by APA and NICE (Chambless et al., 1998; NICE, 2020). It's also a contending treatment for EDs (e.g., Becker et al., 2020) and likely serves as a leading mechanism of action in many successful ED treatments (see Chapter 6).

However, exposure therapy may not work for everyone. Research has shown that while most anxiety and OCD patients experience significant symptom improvement, some may not respond as well or may only partially respond to treatment (van Balkom et al., 2008). Similarly, as discussed in Chapter 6, exposure therapy alone does not appear to be enough when treating EDs (Waller & Raykos, 2019). Reasons for limited success are unclear but may include comorbid conditions, disorder severity/complexity, individual differences, and poor execution (Abramowitz, 2013) (see Chapter 20). To increase effectiveness, this chapter will discuss common mistakes, pitfalls, poor decisions, and challenges for therapists that may impact therapy outcomes.

Mistakes Made in Exposure Therapy

Negative Perception and Apprehension

Exposure therapy has faced criticism and negative perceptions from practitioners (Richard & Gloster, 2007). One could argue that it has a bit of a "public relations" problem. Some practitioners hold negative beliefs about the therapy, such as the idea that it only works in research settings or that it is cruel, which can prevent them from using exposure-based techniques in the treatment of anxiety disorders (Becker et al., 2004a, 2004b; Boudewyns & Shipley, 1983; Fontana et al., 1993). Studies have illustrated that clinicians are often highly anxious during exposure therapy (Schumacher et al., 2014, 2015), which can impact treatment and decisions. Even practitioners who are trained and willing to use exposure therapy may be influenced by negative beliefs about its effectiveness or potential harm

(Deacon & Farrell, 2013). Research by Becker et al. (2004) suggests that clinicians' concerns about exposure causing discomfort or distress for patients can lead to underutilization of this therapy in clinical practice. A survey of more than 600 mental health professionals found that these concerns are common among practitioners from various disciplines, including those who regularly use exposure therapy (Deacon et al., 2013; Farrell et al., 2013). Clinicians may be hesitant to use exposure therapy due to discomfort with inducing short-term distress or misunderstanding the therapy (Harned et al., 2013; Meyer et al., 2014; Parker & Waller, 2017). This can result in not using it at all, or poor implementation (e.g., avoiding high-level exposure, overusing imaginal exposure), leading to less than optimal results.

The gap between research and practice related to exposure therapy in the treatment of EDs is even more apparent. While exposure therapy is not typically used as the primary treatment for EDs directly, there may be an implicit element of exposure in these treatments which may contribute to their strong outcomes (as discussed in Chapters 5 and 6). Many clinicians who specialize in the treatment of EDs may not have as much expertise in anxiety disorders/OCD or exposure therapy, leading to limited training in these techniques. D'Souza et al. (2019) found that the more positive ED clinicians' beliefs were about the value of the therapeutic alliance, the less likely exposure was to be implemented – including challenging eating patterns, weighing, and structured eating (Mulkens et al., 2018).

Clinicians may make mistakes in exposure therapy for EDs due to limited training, exposure to disorder-specific myths, and nonstandardized treatment practices in the United States (Harned et al., 2013; Meyer et al., 2014; Parker & Waller, 2017). For example, the word "fat" has evolved in meaning and connotation, with some groups reclaiming it as a source of pride in the face of its use as a weapon against higher-weight individuals. However, many clinicians working with EDs may reflexively respond to their patients that they are not "fat" if this was expressed. While in some contexts (i.e., CBT, "reality-testing") this response could be appropriate for patients who are objectively thin and experiencing distortions, it can be a missed opportunity for patients to develop a neutral or reclaimed relationship with the word, as well as a missed opportunity for some to tolerate uncertainty related to a fear of weight gain. This response can also reinforce the harmful narrative that being larger is "bad," which has cultural ("fatphobia") and clinical implications (reinforcement of fears). It is important for clinicians to fully understand the conceptualization of the patient's disorder, be aware of their core fears, and have a thorough understanding of exposure therapy in order to optimize treatment outcomes.

Failing to Identify Core Fears

Exposure therapy involves confronting feared stimuli without the use of safety behaviors or avoidance (Kamphuis & Telch, 2000; Powers et al., 2004; Rodriguez & Craske, 1993; Telch et al., 2004). To maximize the chances of successful treatment, it is important to have a thorough understanding of each patient's core fear and the associated feared consequences, triggers and contexts, and avoidance behaviors (Moscovitch, 2009). The EPT model suggests that patients need to process new information that conflicts with their existing fear structures in order to facilitate learning. It is crucial to understand the nuances of a patient's thoughts, emotions, and behaviors as they relate to the fear, and for the exposure to target the precise core fear in order to facilitate new learning.

Consider the case of Mallory, who presents with OCD and reports a range of obsessions and compulsions related to a fear of harming someone. Mallory avoids using knives, prays repeatedly while driving, avoids carrying her baby up and down steps, and avoids taking trains. It can be overwhelming for a clinician to identify and create a treatment plan to address all of the symptoms that are present in a patient with multiple obsessions and compulsions. To streamline treatment, it is important to identify the core fear, which can be thought of as a key card in a house of cards that supports all of the obsessions and compulsions. If the right exposures are chosen based on the accurate core fear, it may not be necessary to address all of the obsessions and compulsions individually for the house of cards to come down.

Identifying the core fear ensures that the items on the hierarchy are all relevant, facilitate new learning, and improve treatment outcomes (Gillihan et al., 2012). If the core fear is misidentified, the patient may not learn new information and treatment may be less effective. For example, if the clinician assumes that Mallory's fear of using a knife to harm her husband is driven by concern about hurting a loved one, rather than a fear of going to jail and leaving her baby with her perceived incompetent husband, the hierarchy of in vivo and imaginal exposures will be less effective. It is important to carefully assess the core fear early in treatment.

Historically, the importance of core fear identification has been known in the treatment of various anxiety disorders (i.e., panic disorder, Salkovskis, 1991; social phobia, Edelmann, 1987; Hofmann & Barlow, 2004). However, it is also crucial in the treatment of EDs. Take ARFID as an example. One of the primary reported reasons for avoiding food is a fear of aversive consequences of eating. Identifying the specific fear (e.g., fear of choking and then dying, or being embarrassed to return to school after a choking incident) can inform treatment and lead to more rapid outcomes. People with other EDs may report a fear of weight gain or changes in their body, but there may be a variety of underlying core fears driving this endorsement (e.g., fear of negative evaluation, loss of social rank or status, loss of romantic partner)

Let's take a look at the case of Connie, who has been undergoing CBT-E for AN. She received traditional interventions and stages of treatment. However, Connie's conceptualization of her disorder included not only an overvaluation of her appearance and a phobic response to food and weight gain, but also a fear of losing her ED. Connie believed that her ED was the only reason people cared for her and that it was what made her interesting; hence, she reported that her fear of recovery was greater than her fear of weight gain. To address this, the treatment plan was modified to include exposures that focused less on the fear of weight gain and more on the fear of being a person without an ED. Connie believed that the lack of an ED would make her boring as a person, and thus she would lose her friends. Therefore, the assigned exposures included telling friends and family that she was recovered from an ED, reminding herself that eating is easier now by getting second helpings of food, gradually reducing assistance from professionals with meal planning and allowing her to choose her own foods, and tolerating the uncertainty that she may be boring and lose her friends if she behaves like a recovered person. Understanding the core fear, or what is maintaining the disorder, is crucial in treatment planning.

Misunderstanding Theory

Many mistakes can be made, as well as opportunities missed, to enhance exposure when a clinician is not well versed in the theoretical basis for exposure therapy.

Explaining Rationale

An untrained therapist may lack understanding of exposure treatment and thus the ability to effectively explain the rationale to the patient early in treatment. It is essential for the patient to understand how exposure therapy works and why it is so important, as the process can be challenging and motivation is a predictor of outcomes. It is also critical to explain the importance of avoiding safety behaviors and rituals in the process. If the patient does not fully understand how exposure works, they may continue to engage in mental rituals or incomplete homework, potentially leading to increased treatment attrition.

Oversimplification

Exposure techniques may seem straightforward and intuitive to many people, especially when the idea of facing one's fears is common in cultural idioms (e.g., "getting back on the horse"; Becker et al., 2020). As a result, inexperienced clinicians may feel confident in simply creating a hierarchy of feared items without considering important elements such as safety behaviors or core fears. Additionally, there is a significant lack of consistency in the standard of training in the field of psychology and in the dissemination of knowledge of exposure techniques (Abramowitz, 2013), and a gap between research and practice. Abramowitz notes that even clinicians and trainees who receive training in exposure therapy often focus more on techniques than on the underlying theory, which can lead to less than optimal outcomes. Therefore, it is important to recognize that exposure therapy can actually be quite complex (Gillihan et al., 2012).

Failing to Incorporate Family and Friends

An inexperienced therapist may not fully understand the importance of discussing the role of family and friends in exposure therapy for OCD. Family accommodation, which is when family and friends cater to or reinforce obsessive thoughts and compulsive behaviors, can perpetuate the individual's OCD symptoms and make it more difficult for them to learn new, healthy coping skills and achieve lasting change. As previously stated earlier in this chapter, high familial accommodation does in fact predict poorer ERP outcomes in children for OCD (Garcia et al., 2010; Storch et al., 2007), but this is also important to highlight for individuals with EDs. Families of ED patients may be placed in situations where the patient constantly asks about portion sizes, their body image, or whether they should feel guilty about certain foods, which can maintain the disorder.

Unique to EDs, families, partners, and friends may also have their own misguided or unhealthy beliefs about food and appearance. We've worked with parents who believe that people cannot be happy in bodies that are not aligned with societal norms. Often, we find that these parents themselves were not happy at higher weights or may have experienced or witnessed weight stigma, including bullying and discrimination. It may be unimaginable that their child could be content in such a body, and, by reinforcing thin ideals, they may believe they are protecting their child from negative consequences. Parents and partners that overempathize with the experience of "feeling fat" may discourage the higher-calorie diets that are sometimes needed to achieve health and weight restoration (see Chapter 7). Taking the time to provide education to families about how these beliefs maintain the disorder, along with assuring families that their loved ones will gain skills to tolerate negativity, is sometimes required to decrease accommodation in the home during treatment. Providing education and training to families can create a more conducive home environment and help prevent compulsions.

Failing to Maximize Inhibitory Learning

According to ILT, fear associations do not disappear during extinction, but rather remain intact while new, more neutral associations with the stimulus are learned (Craske et al., 2008). After a successful exposure, the feared stimulus now has two competing meanings: the original fear-based meaning and a safety-based meaning. These two meanings compete when the individual confronts the stimulus. Because we are wired to remember the "bad" or more scary experiences more robustly (the memory of touching a hot stove will always win), treatment should be enhanced to increase the knowledge and accessibility of the safety-based meaning. One strategy that can be helpful in this process is expectancy violation.

Expectancy Violation

The greater the mismatch between what is expected and the actual outcome, the more the safety-based learning will be enhanced (Craske, 2015). To maximize the violation of expectancy, the therapist can ask the patient to predict in precise language what outcome they expect during an exposure. Testing this expectation can help enhance learning about the feared stimulus and the individual's reaction to anxiety.

Response Prevention, Reassurance, Safety Cues

Learning theory (e.g., Lovibond et al., 2000) also provides a context for the importance of RP. Safety behaviors appear to hinder learning at least in part by interfering with the development of inhibitory associations (Craske et al., 2008). Exposure therapists must be mindful of the creative (and "sneaky") ways their patients' thoughts can lower anxiety levels and covertly maintain rituals. Mental compulsions in particular are tricky because they are unobservable and novice clinicians may miss them or misinterpret them as obsessions (Williams et al., 2011). It may be helpful in preparation to create overt statements to preemptively "spoil" the potential mental compulsion during exposure. In OCD, clinicians should be aware that psychoeducation, including insight statements like "that's just my OCD," can become a mental compulsion (Gillihan et al., 2012). Other cues, such as having a therapist present for exposure or keeping a cell phone in a tight grip, can become a safety behavior and are often missed.

Similarly, reassurance can prevent direct exposure to the feared stimuli. This robs the patient of having to tolerate high distress and learn new information about the stimulus along with their ability to handle anxiety (Abramowitz, 2013). It is often very natural for less experienced, well-meaning therapists to provide constant reassurance, especially given the glaring illogical connections people with OCD and EDs report (i.e., gaining 10 pounds from one slice of pizza). There is some debate regarding the effect of distraction during exposure; however, multiple studies have found that it is most ideal for the patient's full attention to be on the feared stimulus instead of distracting themselves (Grayson et al., 1982). The general consensus in the field encourages clinicians to not distract (Parrish et al., 2008). Overall providing safety, distraction, and other interventions that may "help" the patient get through the exposure can potentially convey a mixed or inconsistent message. You want your patient to feel that you believe that they can do it and that they can tolerate whatever outcome happens.

Removing safety behaviors can be even more challenging in ED treatment. Gold-standard treatments such as CBT-E will actually encourage patients earlier in treatment to use safety behaviors to complete their food goals (i.e., wear baggy clothes, eat whatever food you want regularly). Depending on the target, safety behaviors may be appropriate. If weight gain and increasing caloric intake is crucial for the patient's psychological and physiological well-being, distraction or relaxation techniques could be appropriate early in treatment, as seen in FBT. Clinicians should exercise caution and consider resisting reassurance to ED patients, much like when working with OCD patients. Not only is the world unpredictable and patient fears may sometimes come true (e.g., a boyfriend may break up with a patient after weight gain), their metabolism during ED treatment is unpredictable as well (see Chapter 7). Similar to the needs of anxiety patients, clinicians in ED treatment should refrain from reinforcing messages that anxiety is bad and should avoid providing reassurance for similar reasons regarding weight fears.

Spontaneous Recovery

If a clinician does not understand the theoretical basis of learning, they may not realize that a fear does not simply disappear after exposure therapy. While exposure therapy can reduce an individual's fear, it may still be retained in some form during extinction and may return in certain contexts, a phenomenon known as "spontaneous recovery" (Quirk, 2002). For example, consider the case of Kaitlin. Restaurant exposures were part of her treatment plan. After successful discharge, Kaitlin reported low levels of anxiety for these and related fears. However, six months later, during a booster session, Kaitlin reported significant anxiety around eating outside her home. Due to the coronavirus pandemic, she had been making most of her meals at home. Interestingly, Kaitlin was not in full relapse, as she continued to eat regularly and maintain a routine. It appeared that the natural avoidance of restaurant food was enough for the fear to spontaneously return. This example highlights the distinction between "programmed" exposures, which are deliberately set up in treatment, and "lifestyle" exposures, which are part of an individual's everyday life (Abramowitz et al., 2003). It is important for clinicians to communicate the importance of continued exposure to fears and of incorporating these fears (restaurants) into life "organically" (i.e., socializing).

Overconcern with Habituation

When clinicians are not familiar with the theoretical foundations of exposure therapy, they put too much emphasis on habituation and become concerned when their patients' fears are not reducing (Abramowitz, 2013). While many patients do habituate to their fears, research has shown that some individuals may have deficits which limit habituation (Jovanovic et al., 2010; Milad et al., 2009). It is important to note that habituation is not a necessary condition for extinction learning to occur during exposure (Craske et al., 2008; Rowe & Craske, 1998). While habituation and reducing anxiety may still be important targets in treatment (Becker et al., 2020), inhibitory learning is considered to be central to extinction (Bouton, 1993). Failing to understand the importance of inhibitory learning and focusing too much on habituation may lead therapists to make mistakes or fail to enhance treatment, including a DT focus. Previous research has shown that the affect intolerance constructs (DT, IU, AS) are implicated in the development and maintenance of both OCD and EDs. It has been argued that tolerance of fear, for example, may be more critical than fear reduction in and of itself (Abramowitz, 2013; Berman et al., 2010; Craske, 2008). Exposure to prolonged periods of anxiety may be just as beneficial as exposure to the actual stimulus that evokes the emotion (Eifert & Heffner, 2003). Targeting these clinical features rather than fear reduction may have longer-term benefits in terms including resiliency and relapse prevention.

Inhibitory learning models do not emphasize fear reduction and may even design strategies to maintain high levels of fear throughout exposures. Additionally, because EDs are complex disorders in which exposure alone may not be sufficient and the reduction of anxiety around food is not continuous, focusing only on habituation may limit treatment.

In Summary

Exposure therapy is a well-established and effective treatment for anxiety disorders and OCD. However, it is important to note that like any treatment, exposure therapy may not work for everyone (van Balkom et al., 2008). There are several potential reasons for this, including therapist limitations such as having a negative perception of exposure treatment or not fully understanding the learning theories that underlie exposure therapy. These limitations can lead to implementation deficits in treatment, such as failing to adequately explain the rationale for treatment, missing the core fears, providing too much reassurance or allowing safety behaviors, or not effectively using techniques to maximize inhibitory learning. These factors may contribute to poor outcomes for some patients. Clinicians may need to think outside of the box, using creativity and a trial-and-error approach in order to tailor exposures correctly to improve outcomes.

Considerations for Exposure Therapy in Eating Disorder Treatment

EDs have a significant overlap with OCD and anxiety disorders. There have been arguments to categorize EDs as an anxiety disorder within a larger transdiagnostic model or to view them as a spectrum of disorders (Hollander et al., 2005; Pallister & Waller, 2008). Data strongly indicates that the behavioral elements of treatment (i.e., exposure) generate most of the change occurring in therapy for these disorders (Ougrin, 2011; Parker et al., 2018). Specifically, exposure has been shown to be effective in the treatment of anxiety disorders and in OCD. However, despite the similarities between EDs and anxiety disorders and their respective treatments, there are some differences in the application of and response to exposure therapy in EDs. As mentioned in previous chapters, there may be more allowances for reassurance, safety behaviors, and distraction during exposures to food if the primary treatment goal is weight gain. Additionally, exposure could be affected by starvation and may require a longer process. The ego-syntonic presentation of some EDs can make treatment less volitional and therefore risk the presence of mental rituals or other covert compulsions that can slow down the effects of exposure therapy. There are also disorder-specific factors (i.e., treatment manual avoidance in ED providers) that make the utilization of evidence-based treatments more scarce and lead to differences in application. This chapter will outline these challenges and provide a foundation for solutions found in later chapters. Some of the reasons for poor delivery or treatment manual avoidance are known and documented. These reasons coincide with difficulties seen in the anxiety-based field, which include clinician's attitudes, anxieties, and concerns about evidence-based treatment. We also hypothesize that there are lesser cited and more complicated reasons why evidence-based treatment models are used less in the ED field (i.e., culture).

Clinician Differences

Lack of Training

As demonstrated in Chapter 11, the gap between research and practice in the field of EDs appears wider than in the anxiety disorder domains. There is evidence to suggest that very few ED clinicians use evidence-based treatments, and, even when they do, they do not exercise fidelity to the model. For example, studies have found (Tobin et al., 2007; Wonderlich et al., 2017) that only a small percentage of ED treatment providers reported that they adhere closely to treatment manuals and that employment of such treatments has been delayed or is inconsistent (Wonderlich et al., 2017). Even when clinicians do choose to use an evidence-based manual that includes exposure therapy like CBT, there are often difficulties with delivery and adherence (e.g., Mulkens et al., 2018; Waller et al., 2012).

Highlighting this, Waller (2016) points out that despite growing bodies of literature and numerous protocols to help clinicians provide effective, evidence-based manuals with good outcomes, relatively few clinicians are using them.

Attitude, Concern, Anxiety

Clinicians often hold negative attitudes toward manualized treatments and prefer eclectic or integrative approaches (Waller, 2016). They view manualized treatments as too constraining and lacking the "artistry" of treatment delivery. This can result in using interventions with little or no empirical support (Addis & Krasnow, 2000; Waller, 2009). In addition, clinicians may have concerns about exposure therapy's impact on their patients and the therapeutic alliance, leading to reduced use of exposure therapy in ED treatment (Becker et al., 2004a, 2004b; D'Souza et al., 2019; Meyer et al., 2014). For example, therapists may omit exposures, such as weighing patients, or avoid implementing structured eating, both of which have been shown to be crucial for successful outcomes (Mulkens et al., 2018). Therapists may also be hesitant to use FBT for adolescent AN due to various concerns and challenges (i.e., role reversal, power dynamics, severity of AN, fear of rupturing families, need for more supervision), despite it being the best-supported treatment (Le Grange et al., 2017; Lock & Le Grange, 2008). Last, clinician anxiety while facilitating exposure therapy can lead to a delivery that is more restrained (i.e., not pushing a client further on their fear hierarchy, overusing imaginal exposure). Clinicians are often anxious while facilitating or watching their patients engage in an exposure (Schumacher et al., 2014). This has also been the case for us, and, in our experience, sometimes therapists can catastrophize just as much (or more) than the patients about exposure outcomes (especially around weight). Overall these problems will prevent ED patients from receiving good treatment despite research demonstrating good outcomes.

History of Treatment

The stigma that patients with ED cannot get better is still recent history. This notion once applied to OCD prior to the development of ERP. Although this myth has more recently been publicly dispelled, the stigma still lingers and could contribute to clinicians' lack of motivation to find models that are manualized for ED treatment as they require more intensive training and involve more time and money – why expend the resources when the patient won't get better anyway? Social psychology explains that even when a stereotype has been challenged and successfully shifted, the emotional "feeling" of prejudice associated with that cognition tends to linger. Even clinicians who are aware that the data indicates that individuals with EDs can get better may still "feel" like they are a hopeless population. In this case, one may be more likely to provide supportive talk therapy and life skills to help the patient "manage" the ED rather than seek out and commit to an evidence-based treatment model.

Additionally, as Chapter 8 explained, the historical standard of care for EDs typically involved an outpatient therapist that relied heavily on a dietitian to implement behavioral interventions (i.e., food logs, weighing the patient) and would quickly refer to a residential facility when symptoms increased. The therapist's primary role in this model was to "address the underlying issues," or, in other words, "identify the root cause of the ED." This antiquated model was used for a very long time. Changing this model has implications for business relationships between various different providers, especially those in the United

States with private practices. This may require systemic and cultural change rather than an individual provider shifting a type of intervention (i.e., collaborative versus hidden weights), which takes more energy.

Disorder Differences

Complexity

Beyond the history and traditional treatment possibly accounting for some of the apathy or disinterest in evidence-based treatment, particularly exposure, the complexity of EDs could be another factor.

Danger Risk

The hesitancy many clinicians experience in using exposures for domains such as anxiety disorders and OCD can be higher with EDs. This is likely greater because EDs patients have a high mortality rate, a high self-harm comorbidity rate, and significant physiological comorbidities. Often clinicians report feeling hesitant about showing patients their weight because they fear it will activate not only their patients' anxieties, causing worsened behaviors and more psychological distress, but potential physical harm as well (e.g., orthostasis, arrhythmias) from the increase in disordered behaviors (e.g., restriction, purging, etc.). Typically, the patient's response is often more manageable than the clinician anticipates. Further, as Becker et al. (2020) describes, it is typically better to experience "short-term pain for long-term gain" because weight avoidance is often a factor maintaining the illness for most presentations.

Ego-Syntonic

EDs often present as ego-syntonic, wherein motivation is low and the patient's values (e.g., being thin, eating less, eating healthy foods, etc.) conflict with the goals of effective treatment. Although attrition rates for manualized treatment are typically lower than many clinicians assume in EDs, drop-out can be somewhat higher in practice than in research trials (Waller, 2016). This hesitancy to even engage in treatment, combined with clinicians' fear of their patients dropping out of treatment, may disincentivize clinicians from "pushing" their patients. Clinicians are trained to provide interventions aligned with patient values and to convey empathy and support, rather than to challenge. When providing ED treatment, it is sometimes necessary for patients to engage in behaviors (e.g., eating more processed food) that conflict with their values. The combination of these variables can create a situation wherein the patient does not receive sufficiently robust treatment for recovery.

Other Emotions

Broadly, exposure may not have the same effect that is observed with anxiety-based disorders. There are other aspects of the ED that are unlikely to respond to exposure treatment: constructs found in EDs, including anger, low self-worth, and an identity associated with having an ED, will likely not remit with exposure. This is seen in other disorders as well, including PTSD. For example, Resick et al. (2002) found that although exposure reduced anxiety, cognitive restructuring was found to have a larger effect on other emotions, such as guilt and shame.

Weight Stigma and Cultural Barriers

Many of the core fears and daily hesitations that ED patients experience (e.g., fear of weight gain, avoidance of sweets, etc.) on a pathologic level are uniquely normalized and often are experienced on a less intense, frequent, and impairing level within the greater population and culture. These behaviors can be praised and glorified by society, the healthcare community, and the media. Preoccupation with health, body size, and weight are ubiquitous in Western culture, which affects individual beliefs about body and food (e.g., "good foods" versus "bad foods"). Additionally, Chapter 7 considered at length the continued misconceptions about the association between health and BMI. There is a stigma against certain body sizes and body shapes (particularly higher weights) that can be seen on an individual level (e.g., a child being bullied in school) as well as an institutional level (e.g., health systems misusing BMI). And at the same time, the primary domain in which women invest their self-esteem and worth is that of appearance, which is also growing for other subsets of people such as men (Phillips & Diedrichs, 2015) and the LGBTQIA+ population (DeMarco & Sell, 2015; Reisner et al., 2015).

These societal and cultural beliefs have several reverberating consequences relating to treatment. Many people, including clinicians, may relate to a feeling of discomfort when their weight goes up on the scale (albeit a less intense feeling of discomfort), feeling guilty after eating, or having body dissatisfaction and "feeling fat." Although there are similar tendencies in the general population for other disorders (e.g., concerns about contamination, fear of judgment), weight stigma and valuing appearance is more omnipresent and more deeply rooted in both society and individual self-worth. As a result, a clinician may overly empathize or make incorrect predictions on how a patient may react to a food or weight exposure, which can affect the usage, facilitation, and processing of such exposures. This unique aspect of ED pathology may contribute to the therapist drift (Waller, 2009) in manualized treatments or a complete omission of certain important exposures such as weight exposure.

In addition to the therapist's implicit bias, anxieties, and concerns affecting treatment, the internal experiences of family, partners, and friends can also impact treatment. In Chapter 11 we explore common pitfalls, one of which is failing to educate friends and family early on in treatment to prevent accommodation. Often during treatment for EDs or anxiety-based disorders, well-intended families will provide reassurance, engage in "thought traps" (e.g., "mom, do I look fat?"), accommodate (e.g., cook different dinners for the patient), and undermine the exposure work that the patient is attempting to do in treatment. Many times, partners and parents need their own education, along with DT and ER training, to tolerate and support the patient in treatment. Families can also fall into believing exposure therapy is "cruel" or "harmful" and discourage the patient from challenging themselves. Families may have difficulty watching their loved one experience high levels of anxiety during exposure homework and may encourage the patient to choose a food that causes less distress so they do not have to witness them in distress.

Competing Needs

Although many evidence-based treatments incorporate exposure therapy as a clinical intervention, some ED therapies expose patients to food or scales in a way that is not volitional and typically involves a lot of accommodation early in treatment, and thus it is not considered legitimate exposure therapy. For example, treatments (e.g., FBT) for restrictive disorders (e.g., AN, ARFID) will typically have patients eating foods they are reluctant to eat or making stepping on the scale nonnegotiable in treatment even when the patient reports that they do not want to do it. Although this less-than-voluntary feeding process goes against the principles of how learning happens during exposure, this is necessary at times because of the physical and psychological effects of starvation.

Further, the allowance or suggestion of certain behaviors – such as wearing baggy clothes in CBT-E (Fairburn, 2008), or playing games during meals to distract them from their anxiety and increase eating in FBT – can appear to be safety behaviors. Additionally, clinicians using CBT-E will encourage omitting or delaying eating outside of planned meal times for BN and BED patients, offering coping skills and alternative behaviors to avoid engaging in symptoms. Once the patient has reduced the bingeing behavior, however, the therapist and patient may decide to utilize exposure therapy to learn to tolerate being around and eating these foods without bingeing. These can be useful strategies to change behavior and can help the patient achieve success. It should be noted, however, that these behaviors can easily become safety behaviors which interfere with exposure and weaken the patient's chance of new learning from and gaining full benefit of exposure (Becker et al., 2020). Even though some of these accommodations may be necessary earlier in treatment to foster behavior change and fight the effects of starvation, having an awareness of how these behaviors can become safety behaviors will help facilitate goals later in treatment.

Core Fear Identification

The importance of the core fear was outlined in Chapter 11 and was identified as a common pitfall for clinicians. One of the differences in ED treatment is that the core fear (i.e., gain weight) often needs to come true for recovery, or, at least, there is an increased probability that the core fear might come true (i.e., gaining weight, experiencing weight stigma). Patients who gain weight in treatment may have natural weights or body types/shapes that are more stigmatized in our society, whereupon the goal shifts to tolerating distress of judgment. In OCD and social anxiety treatment, typically the patient's fears are unlikely to be realized. In ED treatment, however, there is a higher probability that some of the patient's fears could come true, thereby complicating treatment. This underscores the importance of inhibitory learning and DT in ED treatment, wherein habituating to fears may not be as applicable and tolerating the uncertainty is not enough. Research has shown that DT is an important factor in the development and maintenance of EDs and other anxiety-based disorders (e.g., Corstorphine et al., 2007). The tolerance of fear and other negative emotions may be more critical to treatment success than fear reduction for a specific stimulus (Craske et al., 2008). It is helpful if the patient aquires skills to manage the outcome of being treated differently or stigmatized over their weight or body shape. The difference in outcome of some exposures may partially account for why EDs take longer to treat and why patients do not respond to exposure treatment quite the same as in other anxiety-based disorders.

In Summary

Exposure therapy can be an effective treatment for both OCD and EDs, but there are some differences in terms of how it is implemented and the outcomes that can be expected for patients with these different disorders. One key difference is that ED therapists may be less likely to use manualized therapies, including exposure treatment, due to a lack of training or negative beliefs about the technique. Another key difference is that EDs are often ego-syntonic, meaning that the individual views their disordered behaviors as a normal and essential part of themselves, while OCD and anxiety disorders are often ego-dystonic, meaning that the individual does not believe that their anxiety is a normal or acceptable part of themselves. Additionally, the emotions and nature of the core fears targeted in treatment may be different (i.e., anger or guilt rather than anxiety). When treating OCD, the focus is on specific thoughts or outcomes, while EDs involve a complex set of fears related to food, body image, and weight. The impact of starvation on treatment and the likelihood of certain core fears, such as the fear of weight gain and experiencing weight stigma, being realized may also differ between the two disorders. It is important for therapists to carefully consider these differences when implementing exposure therapy for OCD and EDs.

Subclinical Features as Treatment Barriers

Given the high rates of co-occurrence between OCD and EDs (Godart et al., 2002, 2003; Halmi et al., 2005; Kaye et al., 2004) and the similarities in presentation and maintenance (Bellodi et al., 2001; Neziroglu & Sandler, 2009; Waller, 2009), clinicians may encounter patients with subclinical features. This can manifest as (1) a primary diagnosis of either OCD or ED with accompanying problematic behaviors such as maladaptive perfectionism and impression management, and (2) a subclinical, yet notable, secondary feature of the other diagnosis. These presentations can pose challenges for clinicians, particularly when patients are unaware of the issues. This chapter will cover these presentations and provide clinical examples. The emerging disorder of orthorexia nervosa (ON), characterized by features of both AN and OCD, will also be discussed.

Perfectionism

One of the most common co-occurring traits to both EDs and OCD is perfectionism (Ashby & Bruner, 2005; Pollack & Forbush, 2013; Shafran et al., 2002; Soreni et al., 2014; Steinglass et al., 2007; Wu & Cortesi, 2009). Perfectionism takes many forms, with some presentations more obvious than others. The most stereotypical and generally straightforward presentation that we see in practice is the profile of high achievement, rigidity, over-preparedness, thoroughness, extreme promptness, and likely to engage in a fair amount of checking behaviors related to many domains and tasks. With regard to EDs, we tend to see this presentation most commonly with restrictive EDs, and with AN in particular. A lesser-known side of perfectionism is the avoidant and somewhat scattered-appearing presentation. This presentation is less recognizable because it can be characterized by underproduction and what looks like carelessness. For example, in the first presentation an individual would have rigid work plans, arrive to appointments early, complete assignments prior to the due date, check to make sure that nothing was missed or forgotten, etc. In the latter presentation, an individual may feel the mental burden of doing these things (e.g., assignments, meeting deadlines) and then engage in avoidance to cope, resulting in late assignments or missing deadlines. Whether the person is aware of it or not, the avoidance is usually related to perfectionistic cognitions. If someone believes that they need to have their whole house clean before they can sit down to start working on the assignment without distraction, they may delay getting started. Paradoxically, they eventually complete the task at the last minute or hand things in late, with mistakes, because of their coping style and perfectionistic beliefs.

In EDs, perfectionism would naturally include content related to diet, eating behaviors, and possibly exercise. An OCD presentation that presents heavily with morality-based obsessions (e.g., "I need to be a good, moral person.") is probably the most vulnerable to having perfectionism extend to food and exercise because of the general stigma and biases surrounding eating, food choices, and exercise in Western culture.

Kathy

Kathy is a 50-year-old woman with long-standing OCD since childhood. Her mother was critical of her throughout her life, often leaving her to believe that she was "not good enough." While this did not cause her OCD, this may explain some of the content of her obsessionality, much of which relates to cleanliness and morality. Her cleanliness presents as compulsions to prevent contamination from dirt and germs (e.g., cleaning objects, handwashing, avoiding touching surfaces prone to germs, etc.). Her morality obsessions relate to being a good, kind, selfless person. As a result, she often goes well beyond the expectation of sacrifice to be a "good person" in the eyes of others. This pattern extends broadly to providing herself to others via money, care-taking behaviors, thoughtful gift giving, and any other behaviors within her ability that might make another person's life easier.

Kathy is also self-critical on a regular basis as she internalized such messages early from her mother. The combination of critical beliefs in addition to a formed association of weight and food choices with indulgence and moral character is where her OCD blends into her eating behaviors. She does not meet the criteria for an ED, but she often restricts her intake and makes her dietary restraint known to others. It is compulsive for her to let people know that she does not eat much dessert and that she would always sacrifice her food if someone else wanted it. The beliefs within her illness are intertwined with fatphobia, whereby she often expresses her desire to maintain a fit, thin frame.

Paradoxically, these comments are sometimes made in front of people who have higher weights and she seems to have little to no awareness that such comments may make people uncomfortable or feel bad about themselves. Kathy would never want to hurt anyone, but her compulsion to make sure others know she is not indulgent and/or careless about her "health" supersedes her need to be viewed as "good" in the eyes of others. However, any evidence that her comments may have insulted someone makes Kathy highly disregulated– she begins to cry excessively, repeatedly stating that she would never want to offend anyone and that she is deeply sorry if her comment conveyed a sentiment of judgment or criticism. The biggest challenge in this case is Kathy's limited insight into the severity of her OCD, particularly the way that it impacts her interpersonal relationships

Impression Management

Impression management refers to the deliberate attempt to manage the other people's impressions of a person, group, or organization. It involves presenting oneself in the best possible light, changing behavior, appearance, and communication to create a favorable image for personal or organizational gain. This can be a conscious or unconscious effort to influence others' perceptions. Most people engage in impression management to some extent, especially in social situations where they want to make a good impression, such as starting at a new school, rushing a sorority, interviewing for a job, public speaking, or going on a date. However, excessive impression management can result in a narrow and inauthentic sense of self and cause anxiety and self-doubt when trying to reconcile true values with societal expectations. This is a common characteristic of individuals with a morality subtype of OCD and those with EDs.

Impression management can impact the manifestation and maintenance of both OCD and EDs. In treatment, honesty with the therapist is an important factor influenced by impression management. To effectively treat these disorders, patients must regularly face and tolerate discomfort and negative emotions during exposure therapy. However, this can be challenging and may lead to noncompliance with treatment goals. In OCD treatment, patients with morality-based obsessionality tend to prioritize being "a good person" over being "a good patient," leading to greater honesty about noncompliance. In ED treatment, noncompliance with meal plans or weight goals is common and may result in a higher level of care due to the serious medical consequences of chronic EDs. Individuals with EDs may distort the truth to appear as a "good patient" to their supports and providers. ED providers are aware of methods patients use to falsify their weight (e.g., water loading, putting weights or objects in clothing). While not the sole reason, impression management is often a factor that sustains dishonesty. This gets especially tricky when a patient has a primary ED with secondary OCD features. Let us consider the case of Grayson to highlight this clinical problem.

Grayson

Grayson is a 21-year-old Asian male in his senior year of college. He and his family have engaged in various treatments for AN since high school (i.e., CBT-E and FBT at different times), and he began to see an outpatient provider when he arrived at college. Grayson struggled with features of OCD, specifically related to exactness and morality. He presented as very bright, academically driven, and as an intellectual at heart. There were some therapeutic alliance challenges, but they eventually developed a nice rapport. With regard to his ED treatment and stability, he voiced motivation to stay at college despite struggling to comply with the recommended caloric intake needed to maintain the necessary weight to do so.

He did not have a history of overtly lying to his parents or his provider in treatment, and although he prided himself on not being dishonest, at times he clearly omitted certain details pertaining to eating. He was able to twist his mind into a pretzel to convince himself that he was not being dishonest. His eating and weight did become more stable while living at home with his parents and doing school and treatment virtually because of the novel coronavirus pandemic. When his school allowed students to return to campus living, specific guidelines were put into place (i.e., weight range) to ensure that he did not regress with his ED. He dropped 4 pounds rather quickly but he understood that this could not continue and was agreeable to developing a plan to ensure stability. Meals and snacks were loosely planned and his weight each week was stable, bouncing back and forth between a 3-pound difference.

Unbeknownst to his provider and his parents, Grayson had actually lost 30 pounds over the course of the semester, not the 4 pounds that was reported. He had held hand-weights at the time that his weight was taken each week. Because of the pandemic, Grayson was unable to attend in-person treatment sessions, nor was he able to go back and forth between school and home for weekends here and there as he had done pre-pandemic. Thus, his parents and provider were limited to only seeing him from the shoulders and up on a computer screen. Whenever questioned if the weight was accurate, he stated that he would never lie about that. Technically, he was telling the truth in reporting the number on the scale, whilst omitting to mention that the hand weights were making his weight register as higher. This is a great example of another twisted "mind pretzel." "Disappointing" his provider by admitting that he had been dishonest is a behavior that is generally viewed as undesirable and conflicts with his beliefs about integrity. In reality, this behavior is related to his pathology, not his moral character; however, the shame and guilt he felt was so high that he was unable to face his provider in a session in order to process it and move forward in treatment.

Primary Disorder with Subclinical Features of the Other Disorder

Another example of this presentation that is not directly impacted by perfectionism or impression management is the case of one primary diagnosis with subclinical features of the other diagnosis. We highlight this with the case of Miriam.

Miriam

Miriam is a 15-year-old high school student who likely had some presentation of OCD since early in childhood that was not detected. When her stress increased due to academic pressures and related obsessionality, she lost her appetite and likely lost some weight. As stated in Chapter 7, malnourishment can have a notable impact on brain functioning, anxiety, obsessionality, problem-solving, and fears related to eating. She did in fact develop fears related to eating, but she was unable to articulate exactly what her fears related to. As a result of anxiety related to eating and weight loss, she began ED treatment but was unable to complete treatment stays due to newly developed obsessions related to swallowing and corresponding compulsions related to chewing without any feared consequences. This not-so-obvious presentation of OCD often resulted in meals not being completed in the allotted time and also frequent episodes of regurgitation that was labeled in ED programs as "purging." Miriam's OCD remained undiagnosed and thus not addressed in all of these rounds of ED treatment, as most ED facilities are not equipped to manage OCD.

Despite these failed attempts at treatment, she did manage to restore some weight and remit fears related to eating. It is notable that she never presented with any degree of clinically significant body image concerns at the onset of her disordered eating or throughout her prior rounds of ED treatment. She entered outpatient treatment with meal completion and fears related to weight loss and "relapse" as her goals. She presented mostly as a high degree of rigidity related to the quality, quantity, and timing of her meals and snacks, in addition to chewing compulsions and regurgitation of food. She was unable to flex at all from the suggested meal plan in residential treatment, even when the food choice was not appropriate to the meal. For example, Miriam would feel compelled to consume a cheese stick on the side of Chinese cuisine because her meal plan suggested having a dairy with meals. She was fearful of relapse in the absence of 100% compliance with her meal plan. She also continued to struggle with meal completion and regurgitation in public due to her obsessions about swallowing her food.

While there is no doubt that Miriam developed disordered eating, her core psychopathology was not consistent with that of diagnosed EDs. Rather, it became clear that OCD was the true primary problem, and that disordered eating and malnourishment manifested as a secondary concern within her broader presentation of OCD. This explains why all of her past ED treatment proved to be unsuccessful. In fact, many of the messages received in such treatment centers (i.e., related to meal completion and "purging") only exacerbated her obsessions and compulsions related to relapse.

ON

In discussing subclinical features of EDs and OCD, we would be remiss to not mention ON. ON is a unique problem in that it is probably the closest presentation to a combination of an ED and OCD. The behaviors are often related to eating and body function, but the content of the fears and obsessionality is what tends to have more of an OCD flare-up (Dunn & Bratman, 2016). It is currently not known whether ON will be included or even mentioned in the next version of the DSM, and, if so, within which category it will fall. Our hunch is that it will be most likely to come under the feeding and ED category; however, OCD may be listed as a differential diagnosis for clinicians to consider.

In Summary

The presentations mentioned in this chapter could present as confusing and perhaps be classified as "treatment resistant" due to some blind spots that may be present when the clinician does not have expertise in both disorders and their related clinical correlates. We suggest that clinicians treating EDs and OCD either singularly or simultaneously ought to remain mindful of the ways in which perfectionism and impression management play out in their patients' clinical presentation and treatment. Similarly, given the high comorbidity rates between OCD and EDs (Swinbourne & Touyz, 2007), whereby simply having this comorbidity decreases the rates of treatment completion for OCD (Kyrios et al., 2015), we suggest a thorough assessment of both disorders (even when patients report a singular chief complaint of one) at the initial evaluation in order to flag any possible secondary subclinical features of the other disorder.

This section aims to provide guidance for best practices to address (and ideally prevent) the previously mentioned pitfalls based on what we have observed in practice and extrapolated from the existing literature. Chapters will provide findings from the literature to suggest why and how some of the interventions in the current treatment protocols could be augmented in cases of comorbidity. The chapters will also include sample dialogue and vignettes from real-life clinical practice (all vignettes have been pseudonymised).

Thorough Assessment

The notion that good treatment with positive outcomes starts with good assessment is not exclusive to OCD and ED. Healthcare providers of all disciplines must create comprehensive treatment plans by combining current empirical evidence for a patient's symptoms and underlying condition, their own clinical judgment, and the patient's willingness to participate in interventions. The success of this process largely depends on the thoroughness of the initial assessment and ongoing follow-up. When treating the complex combination of OCD and ED, it's important to remember that there is no established treatment manual or approach for addressing both disorders. Therefore, a thorough assessment that considers not only the diagnostic features but also the intricacies associated with these conditions is the best guide for clinicians. This chapter highlights some key areas for clinicians to focus on when dealing with this presentation. We hope that considering these variables will better prepare clinicians to tackle this challenge.

Medical Consultation

Perhaps most important when working with an individual with an ED is ensuring their medical stability. This is especially important in outpatient care, where access to physicians/medical care and around the clock monitoring is not feasible. The degree to which medical consultation and ongoing collaboration is warranted will depend on each person's medical presentation, history, and life circumstances. In any event, we certainly recommend that medical consultation occurs at the evaluative stage of treatment, even if further collaboration and/or ongoing medical monitoring are not clinically indicated. A comprehensive review of the medical issues that are associated with EDs is beyond the scope of this book; however, Chapter 7 highlighted some of the most notable issues associated with starvation and low body weight. It is important to keep in mind that a patient's medical stability must be the top priority before beginning any form of outpatient psychotherapy. For example, even if a patient's OCD is severe, as indicated by a high YBOCS score, treatment for an ED should be prioritized if the patient has a low heart rate or low phosphorus levels.

OCD typically requires less medical consultation and collaboration. However, if the patient's obsessions and compulsions are related to a current medical diagnosis, the medical consultation would mainly focus on obtaining unbiased information about the diagnosis from the medical provider. Such information from their medical provider about their condition is useful to form an exposure hierarchy that will trigger OCD while also being objectively safe and free of risk to their safety and health. In addition to informed consent and authorization of information, therapists will explain to patients that their treatment will be based on consultation with their medical provider to ensure that all interventions will be objectively safe. Likewise, clinicians should explain to patients that continued conversations regarding safety are discouraged as this would function as reassurance.

Symptom Timeline

Regarding this co-occurring presentation, it would be helpful to know the timeline of symptoms to help in identifying which symptoms "belong to" which disorder and/or if both disorders have shared symptoms that are difficult to differentiate. In cases where an individual struggles with body image-related concerns in childhood, most EDs have their onset in adolescence or young adulthood. Similarly, with this co-occurring presentation it is most common that OCD or anxiety symptoms were present before the ED (Halmi, 2004). The obsessions and compulsions seen in childhood are similar to those of adults in terms of pattern presentation, but the content of such obsessions differ. For example, many children with OCD have concerns about safety (e.g., a parent dying, being kidnapped), catastrophes, or sources of danger (e.g., natural disasters, school shootings, home invasions). Considering this, it is not surprising that puberty is the time when individuals are most vulnerable to developing disordered eating because this is when the body changes and adolescents start to become aware of social standing as related to their appearance. EDs that present independently or within the context of OCD can often occur inadvertently when an individual is trying to "improve their health" or lose weight.

Having OCD increases the likelihood of developing an ED later in life. For those with childhood disordered eating behaviors and OCD, it's plausible that their disordered eating could evolve into a diagnosed ED later in life. Given the day-to-day rules and rituals of OCD, it would be easy to apply the same patterns to eating. Obsessive-compulsive tendencies increase with malnutrition and starvation, as seen in semistarvation in BN and BED (Fairburn, 2008). In stand-alone EDs, these tendencies occur rapidly and even more intensely when OCD is present. When both disorders are present, symptoms can be difficult to distinguish, and thorough assessment, including questions about symptom onset and changes, can help identify the timeline and core fear. This is important for treatment planning, as some interventions for one disorder may not be appropriate for the other. Identifying the core fear is crucial to designing a treatment plan with effective exposures (see Chapter 11). This is also true for the more insight/values-based interventions done in CBT-E. Let's revisit the case of Margot (previously discussed in Chapter 9) to highlight the importance of identifying the symptom timeline and "diagnostic home."

Margot has obsessions related to food/weight, and also a core fear of becoming a lazy, self-indulgent, unproductive, noncontributive person who only cares about herself. Prior to the onset of her ED, she had strong beliefs in social justice, success, and productivity. However, these concerns became significantly more intense once her ED progressed. The intensity was such that her personality became consumed by these values, resulting in her fixating solely on rules and rituals in order to distance herself from her core fear.

In traditional AN, weight gain is the primary goal regardless of food variety. Many food fears naturally dissipate with adequate weight gain. In the case of Margot, many of her associated fears remained regardless of weight gain because of her core fear associated with "who" she might become. Thus, it was important to focus on specific indulgent foods, such as pancakes, as they were a favorite in childhood. During imaginal exposures, instead of weight gain fears, Margot expressed that because eating pancakes was a voluntary decision, she believed she was a hop, skip, and jump away from becoming a completely vapid, selfish, indulgent person. This is not usually the core fear in AN, highlighting the importance of identifying the underlying fears from the premorbid OCD. This stage in treatment revealed that fears of weight gain and maintaining a healthy weight were not the primary obstacles in the patient's decision to eat normally without instruction from a parent or healthcare provider.

Assessment Measures

Co-Occurring Psychopathology

Clinicians have a variety of measures to choose from for assessment. Overall, we would recommend some type of structured or semistructured clinical interview to assess psychopathology broadly in addition to OCD and ED-specific measures. Measures such as the Structured Clinical Interview for DSM-5 Diagnosis (SCID-5; First et al., 2016) or the Diagnostic Interview for Anxiety, Mood, and Obsessive-Compulsive and Related Neuropsychiatric Disorders (DIAMOND; Tolin et al., 2018) would be suitable for adults and older adolescents. However, the SCID-5 does not contain thorough questioning for EDs or OCD, and for that reason we prefer the DIAMOND. For younger adolescents and children, the DIAMOND adapted for youth is suitable. There is currently a youth SCID for DSM-IV, and the adapted SCID-5 is under development to include parent/guardian reporting features. It is noteworthy that these two measures are only suggested for use for broad psychopathology assessment.

Other disorders to highlight for thorough assessment which are particularly relevant to the OCD-ED presentation are social anxiety disorder (SAD), MDD, substance use disorder (SUD), and PTSD.

SAD

SAD intersects with OCD and EDs relating to patient's concerns about judgments from others along with concerns about eating in public and in social situations (e.g., the food being messy or prone to get stuck in teeth, spillages, etc.), respectively (Kerr-Gaffney et al., 2018). Studies have reported that individuals with SAD are at increased risk for developing EDs, and vice versa. The comorbidity of SAD and EDs is thought to be related to the shared features of both disorders, such as self-consciousness, perfectionism, and fear of negative evaluation.

MDD

Many individuals with OCD and EDs also have co-occurring MDD. Studies suggest that those with OCD have a prevalence of MDD ten times higher than in the general population (Denys et al., 2004); that up to 60–80% of patients with OCD will experience a depressive episode in their lifetime; and that at least one-third of patients with OCD have concurrent MDD at the time of evaluation (Besiroglu et al. 2007; Crino & Andrews, 1996). Because ED and OCD treatment require motivation and behavioral change, careful assessment of depressive symptoms is crucial for patients to comply with treatment recommendations and homework. Likewise, we want to ensure the absence of active suicidal ideation prior to beginning treatment and/or assessment of whether a higher level of care for depression would be warranted.

SUD

Substance use is a notable concern, particularly in EDs. Even when individuals do not have a formal diagnosis of SUD, it is not unusual for individuals with EDs to have a similar approach to substances as they have with food: all or nothing. This is especially relevant in cases of BN and BED, where bingeing is core to an individual's coping style and general approach to life.

PTSD

A diagnosis of PTSD within this comorbidity increases the risk of abusing substances and food, whereby they can function as avoidance and cognitive distraction for painful emotions and memories and result in appetite and weight loss (Mitchell et al., 2021). PTSD can be associated with changes in eating habits, including binge eating and restriction. It is helpful to know whether the disordered eating behaviors stem from PTSD or have been exacerbated by untreated PTSD. It may be useful to plan the order of treatment (i.e., using a separate therapist for PTSD treatment) for the overlapping presentations. Using food or substances excessively can be treatment interfering and a potential safety concern. Let's look at a brief case example to illustrate how untreated PTSD exacerbated both OCD and an ED, even though both of those disorders were present prior to experiencing a trauma.

Carmen

Carmen is a 20-year-old Hispanic college student who has had OCD since childhood. An increased focus on appearance and body image during adolescence developed into an ED (i.e., atypical AN) during high school. Her OCD focused on various domains, one being a focus on morality and integrity. She often found herself preoccupied with thoughts of being a good person and making the most ethical decisions on a day-to-day basis, along with martyr-like beliefs relating to self-sacrifice in interpersonal relationships. While in college she witnessed her close friend die by suicide in front of her. That would be traumatic with a high risk of PTSD onset for the average person, let alone a person with her existing obsessionality. She found herself compulsively recounting the event, analyzing whether she did all within her power to prevent the tragedy. She also began to engage in various arbitrary rituals that made her feel that "others would be safe" in hopes of preventing a similar tragedy with another loved one. OCD and PTSD cognitions joined forces, leading to an unrelenting belief that her mere presence meant that she was responsible for her friend's suicide – thus confirming her obsessional belief that she is not a good person. Her ED began to worsen as she restricted her food to self-punish. She felt that she did not deserve to eat because of "what she had done."

Primary Diagnoses

When assessing for an ED and OCD, the previously mentioned assessment measures do not determine many of the specific symptoms and nuanced features. Similarly, they will not offer much in terms of aiding in treatment planning. Instead, clinicians would be better advised to use measures specifically designed for OCD and ED, such as the YBOCS and the ED Examination Interview or Questionnaire (EDE; EDE-Q; Cooper & Fairburn, 1987). These are not the only measures available to assess the idiosyncratic features of EDs and OCD but they offer appeal. Not only do they have psychometric data (Luce & Crowther, 1999; Phillips, et al., 2014), they are user-friendly and suitable for training new therapists.

Because the EDE (interview) is primarily used in research settings and there are not many clinicians trained in it, EDE-Q, followed by some additional questioning, may be the more practical and time-efficient measure to acquire much of the same data. These measures will allow clinicians to capture the patient's current symptoms in addition to the history of their illness onset and progression over time.

In Summary

The treatment of co-occurring OCD and ED requires a comprehensive approach that combines current empirical evidence, clinical judgment, and the patient's willingness to participate in interventions. Thorough assessment and ongoing follow-up is crucial for the success of the treatment process as there is no established treatment manual or approach for addressing both disorders. Identifying the chief complaint can be difficult due to the overlap of symptoms, and understanding the timeline of symptoms and data from assessment measures is useful, but understanding the specific rituals, rules, and avoided stimuli is the true key to identifying which disorder ought to be targeted more. This chapter highlights some key areas for clinicians to focus on when dealing with this presentation and emphasizes the importance of a functional analysis of the rituals, rules, and avoided stimuli.

Collaborative Conceptualization and Treatment Planning

After gathering important information during the assessment process, clinicians can begin working with their patients to collaboratively develop a conceptualization of the patient's disorder. This early phase of treatment provides an opportunity for clinicians to educate patients about their disorders and obtain informed consent for treatment. It is important for clinicians to conduct a functional assessment of the patient's rituals, rules, and avoided stimuli to better understand the overlap between OCD and EDs. Additionally, it is crucial for clinicians to assess the impact of malnutrition or weight loss on the patient, as this will inform treatment planning and may affect the course of treatment.

Informed Consent

Informed consent is an essential part of any treatment, but it is especially important in the case of comorbid OCD and EDs. There are many factors that contribute to the complexity of this comorbidity, such as the ego-syntonic nature of EDs, the cultural and societal reinforcement of disordered eating behaviors, the gap between research and practice in the field of EDs, and the limited research on how to treat this particular comorbidity. It is important to ensure that patients understand the general expectations of treatment, the boundaries and expectations for remaining in an outpatient setting safely, and that there is no specific manual or set of guidelines for treating comorbid OCD and EDs. It is also important to emphasize that treatment will be collaborative and that the patient will play an active role in shaping their treatment plan. By having a clear understanding of these issues, patients can make an informed decision about whether to proceed with treatment and can feel more confident and empowered throughout the process.

Combined Treatment

We have mentioned in prior chapters that despite the common co-occurrence of EDs and OCD, there is scant information on how to treat the comorbid presentation (Simpson et al., 2013). Because of this, there is no studied and tested manual that clinicians can utilize or follow in practice. Therefore, it should be clearly stated that the treatment provided cannot be considered an evidence-based treatment. Clinicians are able to provide some information on the evidence-based treatments for each disorder, including scientific rationale for interventions, information on treatment outcomes, average length of treatment, etc. Helping patients understand the current status of treatment, including both the limitations for this comorbidity as well as the promising and robust treatments for each disorder, can provide both the information a patient needs to consent.

Treatment Expectations

It is important to discuss general expectations and briefly explain the type of treatment needed in the informed consent process. Many patients who seek treatment for EDs may have the misconception that they can increase body satisfaction without making any dietary changes, that their primary goal should be weight loss, or that they can recover from a restrictive ED without gaining weight. It is crucial to explain to patients that these goals or expectations are not consistent with best practices and may even contradict the very mechanisms of action that are necessary for treatment success.

Additionally, due to the negative public perception of exposure therapy, and the fact that many patients may have long-standing avoidance patterns, it is important to explain the use of exposure early in treatment. Having a clear conversation about the challenge of exposure can be difficult for clinicians because, in some cases, patients may choose not to consent to treatment and may seek treatment elsewhere, or choose not to engage in treatment at all. As a result, clinicians may be tempted to implement a treatment without certain key exposure elements, such as collaborative weighing in the case of CBT-E. Allowing a patient to begin treatment without collaborative weighing is medically risky and it undermines these mechanisms of action, thereby compromising the entire treatment. It is not advisable to continue treatment if, after a number of sessions, the patient cannot consent to all aspects of treatment. Doing so is unlikely to result in improvement and may increase the likelihood of harm, while also decreasing the patient's trust and hope that any treatment can help them.

Medical Expectations and Safety

Due to the complexity of this comorbidity and the potential medical and mortality risks associated with EDs, it is important to set clear expectations for treatment early on, with a focus on medical safety. This includes circumstances wherein higher level of care may be necessary (i.e., irregular lab work, a significant drop in weight, maintaining a low weight for an extended period, noncompliance, suicide risk) and the importance of regular contact with a physician. Informed consent should emphasize that safety is the top priority, and that patients are expected to follow through with doctor appointments and other recommended treatment. The goal is to keep the patient safe and ensure that their treatment is tailored to their specific needs.

Conceptualization

Functional Assessment of Rules, Rituals, and Avoided Stimuli

It is well established that the co-occurrence of EDs and OCD can create complex cases that are challenging to treat. One reason for this complexity may be the overlapping symptomatology of the two disorders, which can make it difficult to distinguish between behaviors that serve one disorder versus the other. Therefore, it is important to understand the underlying thoughts and meanings behind these behaviors in order to inform treatment. A functional analysis, to assess the purpose of the behavior, can provide valuable data for creating a treatment plan. Here we provide some examples of patients who engage in a number of rituals, avoidance strategies, and safety behaviors that could potentially serve either or both an ED or OCD. In the examples, we highlight how analyzing the function of the behaviors helps gain clarity over which symptoms of the two disorders overlap and thus determines which interventions would be most effective. By understanding the root and function of the patient's behaviors, it will be possible to prioritize treatment and develop a promising treatment plan.

Madison

Madison is a 14-year-old female who has been diagnosed with both an ED and OCD. She recently completed inpatient treatment for AN and has been receiving outpatient FBT. Madison has also been referred for further treatment of her OCD. During her assessment, Madison reported engaging in excessive exercise. At first glance, this behavior could be interpreted as being related to Madison's fear of weight gain or as a way to compensate for calories. However, when working with a co-occurring ED and OCD presentation, it is import- ant to ask detailed questions about the behavior and its function in order to accurately understand Madison's symptoms. By conducting a functional analysis and exploring the thoughts and meanings behind Madison's excessive exercise, it will be possible to clarify the role of the behavior in relation to both of her disorders and inform treatment.

THERAPIST: Madison, you reported that you have to exercise every day and you never miss a day, is that correct?

MADISON: Yes, I wake up at 5am every day to work out in the garage before school.

THERAPIST: Wow, 5am? That's early, especially for a teenager. What does the workout look like?

MADISON: I do the same thing every day. I start at exactly 5:01am and I run in place for exactly 29 minutes until 5:30am and then I do arm weights where I need to do 11 exercises on each side.

THERAPIST: I notice you are very routine and exact with this workout; why do you think you've been doing that?

MADISON: Well, I started doing it one day and then I felt like I had to keep doing it. I noticed it felt right and good at the 29-minute mark to stop, so I just kept working out for that long after that. It feels weird or wrong to think about not doing this every day.

THERAPIST: Why did you start working out in the first place?

MADISON: I think it started when I became freaked out about weight gain during the early stages of FBT. I wanted to prevent gaining weight back. I was doing it at 5am so my mom wouldn't find out but I guess because of all the food I was given, I gained weight anyway. I started to feel better about the weight gain a couple months ago, but I still feel like I have to do the workouts.

THERAPIST: It sounds like your weight or what you're eating is no longer motivating your workouts?

MADISON: Yeah. I don't even really feel so motivated to do it anymore at all or care that I exercise. Ever since I gained weight back, I have been feeling better about my body but I still feel like I have to keep my routines. I have a lot of routines that are similar to this one. I have to shower for exactly 7 minutes and I have an order of how I bathe myself. Also, I need to fill my water bottle up when it reaches a certain line on the bottle. I like to keep my water bottle with me at all times.

THERAPIST: Yes, you mentioned a lot of these routines during the assessment. It appears that your exercise is a routine that you keep which is similar to your other routines.

MADISON: Yes, all my routines are things I feel like I have to do no matter what.

THERAPIST: What would happen if I asked you to change your exercise routine?

MADISON: I think I would feel the same if you asked me to change another routine, it wouldn't feel right. One time I had to shower without washing my hair twice because I ran out of shampoo and I freaked out. I think that's what would happen to me if I had to cut my exercise short. It just wouldn't give me the feeling that I am doing the right thing. It would make me irritated and anxious. I would be worried that my day wouldn't go the right way.

THERAPIST: How do you think your day would be affected, or what does it mean that it "wouldn't go the right way?"

MADISON: I like to start the day feeling like things are going just the right way. I imagine things would be off throughout the day, maybe I wouldn't be able to concentrate at school or something. The routines are annoying sometimes but I do like the feeling that I am doing the exact right thing.

THERAPIST: In addition to the day possibly being messed up and your feeling like things don't feel right if you changed your workout routine, would your food be affected that same day?

MADISON: I might think a little more about what I am eating but I don't think my choices would be different. I just feel like maybe I would be more aware but I don't think I would feel guilty.

In this example, Madison's workout routine appears to be more motivated by her OCD than her ED. There are similarities between her exercise routine and other rituals, such as her strict timing for both working out and showering. It is common for patients with EDs to report enjoying the fact that they are someone who works out, as the disorder often involves ego-syntonic behaviors. In this case Madison reports that she does not enjoy the exercise. Madison also adds that her food intake would not change if she altered her workout routine, suggesting that the compulsive exercise is motivated by a desire for a "just right" feeling rather than a desire to control her body size or shape. These points, along with the fact that Madison is denying that her ED plays a role in her exercise routine, suggests that the OCD is a better explanation for her compulsive exercise in this case.

Chase

Chase, a 13-year-old boy, presents with an ED and possible OCD. One behavior Chase exhibits is frequent handwashing. Through a functional assessment of the behavior, data is obtained to help with diagnoses and treatment planning.

THERAPIST: Hi Chase, I want to ask you more questions about your handwashing. Mom says there are certain times of the day and sometimes when it appears unprompted that you have to get up and wash your hands. What motivates you to do this?

CHASE: Yes, I wash my hands when I feel gross.

THERAPIST: Can you explain what you mean by gross?

CHASE: When there is something on my hands, I feel gross. It happens after I eat.

THERAPIST: What is the primary concern about having something on your hands?

CHASE: Well, I feel like if I don't get the substance off my hands, I am reminded of the food that I ate and it makes me feel even more guilty, fat, and gross.

THERAPIST: So, during eating or maybe after eating, if food is on your hands, you feel like you need to wash it off to prevent thinking about the food later and avoiding guilt?

CHASE: Yes. I was eating pizza the other day and my mom wouldn't let me blot the pizza. I was forced to eat it with all that grease on it and some of the grease got on my hands. It feels gross because then I am thinking about the grease I ate which is definitely going to make me so fat. I want to wash it off as soon as possible and just try to forget about lunch altogether.

THERAPIST: Is there any concern about absorbing calories through your hands or washing your hands to prevent any other contamination like sickness?

CHASE: No, I don't really think about that. It's just so painful for me to remember that I ate food at all, but especially greasy things or things that are sticky because that means that the food had sugar in it.

THERAPIST: It sounds like remembering what you've eaten is very painful for you, is there anything else you do to try to avoid the idea that you consumed food or certain types of food?

CHASE: Yes, I brush my teeth right after a meal if I'm home. If I can't do that, I keep mints or gum with me so I can forget the flavors of the meal and think about the food less.

At first glance, Chase's frequent handwashing and toothbrushing may seem like a sign of a desire to prevent contamination or a compulsive cleanliness routine. However, further assessment reveals that these behaviors are related to his ED. It appears that Chase is engaging in safety behaviors in order to reduce anxiety and guilt after meals. This suggests that the underlying motivation for his handwashing and toothbrushing is related to his ED rather than a separate issue such as OCD.

Amir

Amir, a 22-year-old non-binary college student, seeks an assessment after losing a significant amount of weight due to restricting their intake to mostly fruits and vegetables with some carbohydrate products. They also report having a lot of anxiety and behaviors related to contamination fears and fears of sickness, as well as moral concerns. A diagnosis of OCD was provided based on the time, distress, and compulsions Amir experiences related to contamination and morality. Additional functional assessment of their eating habits was discussed to further investigate their clinical presentation.

THERAPIST: Amir, in the beginning of the assessment we discussed how you have intrusive thoughts about morality as well as getting sick. You explained that the thoughts have become obsessional and in order to prevent sickness or feeling like a bad person, you engage in a lot of compulsive behaviors. I also need to ask you more about why you restrict your intake. What was the first thing you found yourself avoiding eating and why?

AMIR: I have always had a lot of guilt about things and finally one day I said that I have to stop eating animal products because it completely makes me feel like a bad person. If I think I accidentally ate something from an animal, I immediately say a prayer, even though I am not even religious!

THERAPIST: I see. And from our earlier conversation, I noticed you don't eat most fat or protein or really any processed food. What is your reason for that?

AMIR: Well, I cut out animal products to stop feeling like a bad person but then I started cutting out any processed foods because they are not good for your health. I am always checking on my heart rate; I have a lot of fears about getting sick and dying young. I just thought I would eat really clean to stay healthy.

THERAPIST: Okay so you cut out animal products and then you wanted to avoid processed foods, but I see here you avoid all fats and even plant-protein. Does this mean nuts and soy?

AMIR: Yes, I don't even trust plant fats; I am so scared it will clog my arteries. Also, I once read on a message board about how soy protein can mimic estrogen in the body. I'm scared this will increase my risk for breast cancer so I've been avoiding a lot of soy proteins too.

THERAPIST: Amir, do you believe that you try to control the amount of what you eat or just what types of foods you eat?

AMIR: I don't like to have large portions because I know being overweight can cause heart disease. I check food labels constantly to read ingredients but I never really check for calories.

THERAPIST: Would you say that you fear gaining weight or becoming fat?

AMIR: I have become even more scared of weight gain in the last two months despite knowing my weight is too low right now. I never had bad body image before and I always liked my body. It's really weird how I am more self-conscious of my body now and have become one of those people who tries on a million outfits before I go out with my friends. I am afraid of becoming obese because I don't want to die but now, I'm more self-conscious about my body even though I've lost all this weight. It's so confusing.

Although Amir checks food labels and significantly restricts their food intake, it appears that they are motivated by fear of negative consequences such as heart disease and cancer from eating certain foods. This suggests that a diagnosis of ARFID, rather than AN, may be more appropriate. Their ARFID seems to be part of a larger pattern of obsessions and compulsions related to sickness, disease, and morality. Additionally, Amir is beginning to develop body image obsessions and concerns about their appearance due to weight loss. While they did not initially report body image concerns as a motivation for changing their intake, they are now becoming more fearful of weight gain and more concerned with their appearance. From a diagnostic perspective, Amir may soon meet the criteria for AN sequelae weight loss due to their ARFID as well as their morality-based OCD.

Understanding the Overlap in Symptom Presentation

The functional assessment of behavior plays a crucial role in diagnosis, conceptualization, psychoeducation, and treatment planning for co-occurring disorders. It is important to determine whether the disorders are independent or interdependent, and whether they interact with a synergistic quality. Comorbidity often involves some degree of overlap and interconnectedness between disorders, with one disorder often exacerbating the other. For example, a person with ADHD may experience difficulties with school or social interaction, leading to self-criticism and a defectiveness belief which can culminate in a major depressive episode, furthering inattention and focus deficits. In this case, the two disorders are feeding off of each other and present interdependently. On the other hand, someone who has attention deficit hyperactivity disorder ADHD but maintains effective coping skills and does not internalize their focus issues may still experience depression due to external events (i.e., break-up, death); however, their depression is unrelated to their comorbid ADHD. In the comorbidity of OCD and EDs, we may see independent or interdependent presentations.

Independent Presentation

An independent presentation is when the two diagnoses are co-occurring but do not appear to be connected or to exacerbate each other in any way. Arguably, there may always be some element tying the two disorders together, given the genetic relationship or neurological similarities between both disorders. However, despite this phenomenological overlap, some cases may still present without much interaction. Let's look at the case of Alex to illustrate this presentation.

Alex

Alex is a 35-year-old female teacher who presents with both an ED and OCD. Alex reports having struggled with body image issues throughout her life, but her ED behaviors only became significant recently. She states that about 12 months ago, after her fiancé cheated on her, she decided to severely restrict her caloric intake in an attempt to change her body and become more "appealing" when dating. For the past seven months, Alex has been consuming approximately 1,000 calories per day, which she tracks using a fitness app. Despite this significant restriction, Alex has only lost 12 pounds, and currently weighs 160 pounds at a height of 5'4". She avoids desserts and tries to focus on high-vegetable and high-protein meals, and has passed out twice in the last month due to malnutrition. Alex is extremely fearful of gaining even one pound back and weighs herself daily, perceiving herself as "huge" in the mirror. Her friends have shared observations that she has lost weight but she is unable to see this change. She is afraid to go out socially and avoids restaurant food because she panics before eating, which she reports as quite bothersome and distressing.

Alex also reports a long history of anxiety, including OCD since childhood. Recently, Alex has become fearful of becoming sexually attracted to one of her students, causing her to consider changing jobs. She has also experienced panic attacks about the prospect of returning to school and now avoids children. Alex is seeking therapy to address her OCD and receives support for her ED.

In this case, Alex meets the criteria for OSFED, specifically atypical AN. She meets all the criteria for AN, except that her body weight is not considered underweight for her height. Alex also meets the criteria for OCD as she has a history of obsessions and compulsions that have caused impairment and is currently extremely distressed by intrusive thoughts relating to pedophilia. While it is possible that Alex has a genetic predisposition for both disorders, the symptomatology of the disorders does not appear to be interacting. Alex's OCD and anxious presentation has been long standing and does not involve food, health, or rumination with numbers or measurements. Her ED appears to have started from body dissatisfaction and a stressful event that led to calorie counting and food restriction. Overall, there is not much interaction between the two disorders, indicating an independent presentation.

Interdependent Presentation

An interdependent presentation of two disorders refers to a situation where one disorder increases the likelihood of the other, one disorder complicates treatment of the other, one disorder serves as a coping mechanism for the other, and/or the two disorders fuel or exacerbate one other. This type of presentation can be challenging to treat as it may be difficult to identify the functionality of certain behaviors, the disorders can complicate each other, and typical interventions for one disorder may contraindicate the other. Some examples of patients who met criteria for both disorders with an interdependent presentation are given here.

Gary

Gary is a 48-year-old male project manager who works from home and is married with two children in college. He reports binge eating 3–4 times a week and was been diagnosed with OCD many years ago. Gary describes obsessing over things related to his children, his job, and the fear of hurting others. He has a history of seeking reassurance from his children's pediatrician, checking their whereabouts on phone locating apps, and engages in a lot of rearview mirror checking while driving. Since the pandemic, Gary has decreased his driving, which has resulted in increased fear and a decrease in socialization, impacting his mood. He is also worried about offending people at work and has avoided promotion for fear of having difficult conversations with employees.

Gary has been in therapy for his OCD on and off since his thirties, and has found supportive talk therapy to be helpful in coping with his symptoms, but felt best when his therapist would tell him how unlikely it is to run over someone with your car. Despite feeling better after some therapy sessions, he states that his anxieties never went away. More recently, his anxiety and obsessions have been activated even more due to the pandemic, leading him to turn to food as a way to cope with (and numb) his negative feelings. He reports eating large quantities of food in a short period of time as if he is in a trance, multiple times a week, when his anxiety was high over the last year. Gary expresses feeling shameful and frustrated by these habits and is worried about his health. His doctor has commented that he is concerned about his heart health. He tries to skip meals to reduce his calorie intake, but is still bingeing.

In this vignette, there does not appear to be a synergistic effect present; however, the two disorders still have a relationship. It appears that Gary is using binge eating to cope with the anxious or negative states brought on by his long-standing OCD. This example is comparable to the case of Hanna that was given in Chapter 10.

Susan

Susan is a 65-year-old, female, retired accountant who is married with two adult children who live outside of the home. She meets the criteria for AN, which has had a gradual onset since she lost 15 pounds in her fifties. Susan has always had intense body dissatisfaction and reports that thinness and overall appearance were highly valued in her childhood home. Since retirement, she has lost another 25 pounds, putting her at 85 pounds at 5"3." She eats very small portions until dinner and avoids desserts or any "junk" food, but denies that her weight is problematic.

Susan also lives with obsessions around perfection. She is a self-proclaimed perfectionist and goes to great lengths to make everything around her fits into her idea of perfection. This includes waking up at 4am every morning to begin cleaning and doing the laundry, maintaining a strict order of housework, despite not having children in the home anymore, and needing to walk at least 20,000 steps each day in order to feel "complete." She cleans the house for about two hours in the same order every day. Susan describes her house as needing to look immaculate and perfect. She also requires that her food be presented in a certain way and will sometimes throw out an entire plate of food if it doesn't look "nice." She admits that these rituals can be exhausting and that skipping meals because the plate of food doesn't look good enough may be a silly thing to do. Susan feels good when her house is clean and her life is "put together," but she can be envious of her daughter and friends who have more flexibility.

Susan's pursuit of perfection appears to be driving many of her behaviors and habits, and is even impacting her eating. She meets the criteria for both OCD and AN, and her compulsions around needing to attain a certain number of steps and having her food presented in a certain way appear to be driven by her OCD. These compulsions create barriers for weight gain and consistent eating, and therefore the symptoms from the comorbid disorders are interdependent. While the presentations are all different in terms of the idiosyncratic nature of the symptoms, Susan's interdependence is comparable to Margot's OCD-AN diagnosis mentioned in Chapter 9 and Grayson's AN-subclinical obsessive-compulsive features presentation mentioned in Chapter 13.

Sam

Sam is a 22-year-old, female, first-year medical student who lives with roommates. She has been told she is "overweight" by doctors throughout her life, despite having a consistent growth chart since infancy and having parents with higher weights. Sam identifies as always being on a diet and has been bingeing and purging a couple times a week since her junior year of college. She also meets the criteria for OCD and avoids knives or anything that could be used as a weapon due to fear of hurting someone or stabbing them. Sam avoids the kitchen entirely due to intrusive thoughts of stabbing her roommate or bringing a knife to school, and is also afraid of needles in clinical settings. This avoidance of the kitchen has reduced Sam's ability to cook for herself. She also obsesses over money. This leads to shopping avoidance and prevents her from picking up groceries or ordering food regularly. As a result, Sam often goes all day without eating much and sometimes will eventually order food. Because she is so hungry at this point in the day, she often orders a lot, setting herself up for bingeing.

Sam's OCD and ED are closely interconnected. Her anxiety about spending money and harm-based OCD has disrupted her regular eating patterns and increased the likelihood of binge eating. By using Socratic questioning and a functional assessment, the clinician can gain a better understanding of the nature of Sam's disorders and symptoms, which will help inform the development of a treatment plan that integrates evidence-based practices and aims for recovery.

Treatment Planning

After understanding the function of the patient's behaviors and the extent to which different disorders are interacting, treatment can begin. The first symptoms to be targeted should be those that pose a medical impairment or increase mortality risk. For example, if a patient is bingeing and purging so frequently that they are at medical risk, this should be the first symptom targeted, regardless of the patient's potential distress or desire to work on their OCD first. Similarly, if a patient is avoiding spending money on food and therefore restricting intake and increasing their medical risk, challenging these obsessions and compulsions should be the first target, regardless of other less influential dietary rules. This is important to reduce medical and mortality risks, as well as to improve the effectiveness of exposures and CT, which can be less robust in a semi- or full starvation state.

Another factor to consider when deciding which behavior to target first is whether there is clear evidence of one disorder being used to cope with another disorder, as explained in Chapter 10. For example, if a patient with OCD uses binge eating to cope with the stress and exhaustion caused by their OCD, addressing both at the same time may be necessary. Or, in the case of Hanna (see Chapter 10), she was able to prevent bingeing (as an escape behavior) while doing exposure homeworks and allowing for the successful treatment of her OCD. Her OCD remission then allowed for CBT-E for her residual binges. Thus, her BED was treated after her OCD. Clinicians should help the patient understand their ability to overcome binge eating as a coping mechanism, even when triggered. Regulating their diet and using ERP can decrease the frequency of binges. Additionally, it is crucial to provide alternative coping skills to prevent binge eating from becoming the default response to stressors.

Similarly, for a patient with perfectionistic rules and rituals around food that contribute to their restriction, increasing caloric intake may be the first goal. Allowing the patient to continue some of their rules or keep a "perfect" plate at first may help them stay engaged in treatment. If the patient is able to increase their caloric intake even with some rigidity, the weight gain may improve their obsessional thinking, which will be helpful when addressing the OCD. In cases where fears such as spending money is a barrier to meeting the goal of regular eating, ERP may need to be included in the early stages of treatment to allow the patient to increase their food intake. In all these cases, regular eating, along with identifying and targeting any barriers or fears that prevent these goals, will likely be prioritized. Psychoeducation, MI, meal planning support, and self-monitoring records, as well as emotional regulation skills and alternative coping skills, along with ERP and value shifting, will all be provided in the order of need based on the individual's conceptualization.

In addition to understanding what disorder and which clinical features to prioritize, it is important to understand that the priority of disorders and clinical features may change as symptoms can overlap or exacerbate one another, and obsessional content can shift during treatment. For example, Amanda, whose case is outlined here, came to treatment for AN but had a history of OCD. Although her AN treatment was initially successful, her symptoms shifted, requiring a change in treatment plan

Amanda

Amanda is a 32-year-old white female with a history of OCD since early childhood. She also has a history of AN since adolescence that occurred somewhat preceding weight loss due to a medical illness. She continued to have some degree of AN throughout the rest of her adolescence and young adulthood but never received formal treatment (i.e., FBT). She sought ERP at some point in her twenties to address OCD, which she stated was quite effective; however, she also mentioned that she had noticed a pattern of worsened OCD symptoms at points in her life when her weight was lower (pre- and post-ERP). She was also insightful to the fact that eating and the associated preoccupation with food and weight are much less problematic when her weight is higher.

Finally, in her early thirties she decided to seek formal treatment (CBT-E) after losing a fair amount of weight from a worsened bout of AN after the birth of her child. At the start of treatment, AN was very much the main concern due to her low body weight and her preoccupation with food and body image. Therefore, increasing calorie intake and weight gain were prioritized, and she successfully gained 10 pounds over the course of a few months. Based on her prior history of symptom intensity, the goal for weight gain was set at 15 pounds. As she approached this goal, her eating behavior improved, but she still struggled with mental preoccupation with food planning, calorie counting, and concerns about how loved ones perceived her eating habits. She gained some weight and eventually observed that her fears around weight gain and body dissatisfaction had decreased. Instead, she found that her preoccupation with being exact about her daily caloric intake and needing to have a "perfect count" impeded her progress. She also compulsively made announcements to her loved ones about the food she was eating and whether or not the other person "should" have the food instead of her. She was very aware that this behavior was annoying to others and made meals awkward, but the words blurted out of her mouth almost involuntarily. Much of this compulsion boiled down to her obsessionality about others viewing her as indulgent and therefore lazy.

(Note that there is a theme in the obsessionality mentioned for many of these OCD-ED overlap cases, fears of indulgence, and laziness which target the morality domain of OCD.)

It became apparent in Amanda's treatment that while AN was still present, OCD had become the primary concern. The focus shifted from monitoring food intake and weight to preventing rituals associated with calorie counting and announcing food choices, as well as exposing her to eating in front of people who knew about her illness and asking for indulgent foods. Amanda struggled to prevent calorie counting entirely because it had become so automatic. However, the goal was to stop writing it down to avoid formal tracking of daily intake, and to interrupt or "spoil" the counting when she caught herself doing it. Her fears of eating indulgent foods in front of people was related to obsessions about "being a hypocrite." She feared that people who already knew about her history with AN would form judgments about her, as opposed to new people who did not know about her history. This was further evidenced by the fact that she did not make food announcements in front of strangers or newer people.

This example highlights the tricky nature of the presentation and the need for continued reassessment throughout treatment. Without continued reassessment of maintenance variables, a clinician may have continued with self-monitoring, which transitioned into functioning as a compulsion within OCD that also served as a barrier for her gaining the last five pounds needed for her AN recovery.

In Summary

Conceptualization and treatment planning are important steps in the treatment of ED-OCD. During this phase, clinicians work with patients to understand their disorder and obtain informed consent for treatment. Clinicians should conduct a functional assessment of the patient's rituals, rules, and avoided stimuli to understand the overlap between OCD and EDs. Understanding the core fears and functions of the behaviors is also important. Additionally, it is crucial to assess the impact of malnutrition or weight loss on the patient as this will inform treatment planning and may affect the course of treatment. In treatment, priority should be given to symptoms that pose a medical impairment or increase mortality risk, and the overlap of different disorders should be addressed if necessary. In the early stages of treatment, the focus should be on increasing volume of food intake rather than variety. Barriers and fears related to regular eating and weight restoration, such as perfectionistic beliefs, should be identified and addressed. If OCD symptoms (e.g., extreme rigidity or fear of spending money) will directly impact the success of regular eating, these should be addressed using ERP if necessary.

Key Considerations

- Assess the severity and complexity of the patient's OCD and ED, and determine the appropriate level of care.
- Consider the function of the patient's behaviors and the extent to which the disorders are interacting.
- When deciding which behavior to target first in treatment, prioritize symptoms that pose a medical impairment or increase mortality risk, and consider the extent to which the disorders are interacting.

- If one disorder is being used to cope with the other, addressing both at the same time may be necessary.
- Target volume over variety in the early stages of treatment.
- Identify and address any barriers or fears that prevent regular eating and weight restoration, including perfectionistic beliefs or behaviors that may contribute to the ED.
- If OCD symptoms (such as extreme rigidity or fear of spending money) will directly impact the success of regular eating, address these with ERP first if necessary.
- Understand the core fears and the function of the behaviors.

Navigating Meal Planning

Chapters 16–19 provide recommended procedures for addressing and preventing issues in treatment for comorbid EDs and OCD. These are based on observations in practice and in the existing literature. The literature findings will be used to justify potential modifications to current treatment protocols for this comorbidity. This chapter specifically examines the complexities of meal planning interventions for the overlap of EDs and OCD.

Most evidence-based treatments for EDs include guidance on meal planning, as it is widely understood that disordered eating habits or starvation contribute to the core pathology of EDs. As discussed more thoroughly in Chapter 13, OCD can exacerbate ED pathology and make treatment more complex, or, in some cases, ED treatment can exacerbate OCD. Generally, clinical features of OCD such as rigidity, perfectionism, intolerance of uncertainty, and reassurance seeking can disrupt typical ED interventions such as meal planning. In cases of OCD involving food-related obsessions or restriction due to ARFID or ON, certain foods may be targeted or added to a hierarchy, which can also complicate meal planning. Additionally, the content of a patient's obsessions in OCD can shift to different categories in their life, including ED recovery, wherein recovery often becomes a meaningful or central issue. ED treatment can be very intense, taking up a lot of the patient's time, and in the psychoeducation or MI stage the patient spends a lot of time building up the motivation required to overcome their ED. This will inevitably increase the value or meaning of recovery and therefore increase the likelihood that the patient's obsessions will involve ED recovery (e.g., intrusive thoughts that they are going to relapse). We saw this illustrated in Chapter 13 with the case of Miriam. The following sections will provide suggestions for addressing these complications when using meal planning in treatment for EDs and OCD.

Bulimia and BED

Chapter 2 thoroughly examined the leading evidence-based treatments for EDs and found that CBT-ED (i.e., CBT-E and CBT-T) is an effective treatment for BN and BED based on a large body of empirical evidence and positive outcomes. Although FBT has shown to be more effective than CBT-E in some studies on adolescents with BN, CBT-E is still a commonly used and recommended treatment option for adolescent BN (as per NICE guidelines). Chapter 2 also explained how CBT-E treatments aim to shift eating habits to address three main issues: (1) counteracting the excessive focus and value on appearance, weight, and food choices; (2) avoiding the negative effects of undereating, such as emotional dysregulation and increased susceptibility to binges; and (3) challenging distorted beliefs about the impact of certain foods on the body and weight. Some interventions included in

CBT-E for meal planning include eating regularly (every 2–4 hours, based on nutritional needs), planning meals and snacks, working on a hierarchy of feared foods, and involving the patient in food preparation to help meet these goals.

Turning Guidelines into Rules

In clinical practice, we have observed that patients with comorbid OCD may become rigid and perfectionistic about meal planning interventions. They may have difficulty being flexible with meal times and may use meal prepping as a way to control their environment, leading to intolerance of uncertainty. For patients who fear weight gain or changes in their body, rigid meal planning or eating every four hours can provide reassurance about their fears (e.g., "I probably didn't gain weight today because I ate the same thing as yesterday"). In Chapter 13, we met Miriam, who was rigid in ensuring that each meal met all the "required" food groups. For example, she would add a cheese stick to her Chinese cuisine to fulfill the "dairy requirement" even though mozzarella cheese is not typically found in Chinese cuisine and a non-ED person may not consider it necessary to add dairy to this type of food. This illustrates that her rigidity is still present. Some patients may also develop obsessions related to the fear of relapse, such as a sensitivity toward or intolerance of hunger because they have previously binged when feeling hungry. Developing the habit of eating regularly and planning meals can be helpful in reducing binges, but in individuals with increased obsessionality these behaviors may become obsessive and compulsive.

Clinicians should be aware of the potential risks of these interventions for patients with comorbid OCD and EDs. It may be helpful to educate patients about these susceptibilities and involve them in monitoring for obsessionality. To prevent rigidity from taking hold, interventions may be preemptively designed or altered to "shake things up." By this we mean intentionally throwing off the schedule or the plan for eating before the rigidity even starts. For example, a patient who has had a reduction in ED symptoms and success with meal planning every four hours may benefit from eating a few minutes before or after the planned meal time after significant reduction in ED symptoms. Similarly, patients who have been strict with meal prepping may be encouraged to go one meal, then a day, and eventually a week without knowing what they will eat until mealtime and therefore making more planned decisions in the moment.

The purpose of "shaking things up" is not to provide a shift so great that you actually set your patient up for a lapse, but to provide just enough of a shift to act as an exposure that activates a particular obsession (e.g., "if I don't plan every single thing I eat today, I will definitely binge and purge"). While the goal is to use exposure when the patient appears ready (e.g., ED symptoms have reduced), just like in other examples of ERP, the patient should be encouraged to tolerate the uncertainty that relapse may happen. This can be challenging for the clinician, who may also have emotional investment in the outcome of treatment and a desire to prevent relapse. It's important for the clinician to remember that if an exposure or change in meal planning (e.g., eating at 12:15pm instead of the usual 12pm) does significantly derail the patient, this should be viewed as important data and used to improve treatment in the long term. If a 15-minute difference in meal time confirms the patient's binge fears, it may indicate that their recovery is fragile and it is important to catch this early in treatment.

Here are some suggestions for reducing rigidity, perfectionism, and intolerance of flexibility in meal planning for patients with EDs and OCD in CBT:

- Encourage flexibility with a variety of foods: Rather than following a strict meal plan, encourage patients to incorporate a variety of foods and allow for flexibility in their meals. This can help reduce perfectionism and the need for strict adherence to a specific plan.

- Promote flexibility with meal times: Encourage patients to be flexible about meal times and not adhere rigidly to a specific schedule. This can help them tolerate uncertainty and reduce their need for control.

- Encourage flexibility with meal prepping: Rather than always doing their own meal preparation, encourage patients to try going out to eat or having someone else prepare meals for them. This can help them tolerate uncertainty and reduce their need for control.

- Promote mindfulness and self-compassion: Encourage patients to practice mindfulness and self-compassion when meal planning. This can help them be more accepting of flexibility and less rigid in their thinking.

- Help patients challenge rigid thinking: Use cognitive techniques such as cognitive restructuring to help patients identify and challenge their rigid and perfectionistic thinking around meal planning.

- Encourage gradual exposure to flexibility: Gradually expose patients to increasing levels of flexibility in their meal planning. This can help them learn to tolerate and manage their anxiety about deviation from their usual meal plan.

- Use a collaborative approach: Involve patients in the meal planning process and encourage them to take an active role in decision-making. This can help them feel more in control and less rigid in their thinking.

Restrictive EDs

Adolescent Care

Chapter 2 explained that FBT is the leading evidence-based treatment for adolescents with AN, with a focus on weight gain facilitated by the child's parents or guardians. Because AN and its associated clinical features (e.g., obsessionality, rigidity) can be largely attributed to starvation, the child/adolescent is not considered capable of making sound decisions about food. FBT empowers parents to become agents of change in their child's illness and to view their child's thoughts and behaviors related to AN as a symptom of the illness, separate from their child.

The process of increasing food intake and weight in someone with AN can be challenging, and we have observed a potential activation or exacerbation of OCD during this treatment. This may be due to the inherent nature of the treatment (e.g., nonvolitional, intense, loss of exercise), the difficulty of refeeding, or strategies that parents use in treatment (e.g., cooking the same meals, sharing or not sharing calorie counts). This involuntary turnover of control in multiple aspects of life understandably leads to heightened anger, sadness, and anxiety for many adolescents with AN. We have seen a pattern in our patients with comorbid OCD or subclinical obsessionality whereby the patient's rigidity and obsessionality does not reduce simply with weight gain, unlike the obsessional presentation seen in AN. These patients do not achieve the same outcomes as their non-OCD counterparts, according to studies on the effectiveness of FBT (Lock & Le Grange, 2019). Lock & Le Grange (2019) suggest that there may be an opportunity to improve FBT to better accommodate the needs of this comorbidity. Based on our clinical experiences, we have identified behaviors of parents during FBT that could serve as hypotheses for this moderating variable, and we provide the following suggestions for sidestepping these issues in meal planning.

Providing the Same Meals or Snacks

Some children and adolescents with AN, depending on the intensity and duration of the illness and the individual's biology, may become extremely hypermetabolic due to restriction. This means that parents may need to provide densely caloric meals and snacks frequently throughout the day to achieve even moderate gains. In some cases, it may be appropriate to feed the child something almost every hour of the waking day. Due to this demand, along with the other daily demands of parenting, parents may fall into the habit of feeding the child the same thing almost every day. For example, if a parent sees weight success during a week where they provided a child with a CLIF bar and whole milk for the mid-morning snack, a peanut butter and jelly sandwich with potato chips for the afternoon snack, and a tall milkshake before bed, and the child was reasonably accepting of these foods, the parent may stick with these snacks for several weeks.

This consistency may be perfectly reasonable for the average patient. It is likely that their clinical features of obsessionality will reduce naturally with weight gain. Often the types of food accepted will become more varied as the child enters stage two of FBT and lives a more typical life for their age. However, in observing our patients with OCD comorbidity, this has not always been the case. Because the patient's obsessionality is due to OCD rather than AN, they may become overly dependent on or rigid regarding these specific daily snacks. Because of their tendency to use compulsions (e.g., mental reviewing), their fear does not become generalized and opportunities to practice DT are limited. Patients with OCD are more likely to have rituals in general and eat the same thing, which can lead to rigidity despite success with weight gain. Considering the demands placed on a parent during this process and how exposure can help with obsessive-compulsive features, we suggest that even small, realistic changes can help reduce rigidity and the potential reassurance or safety effects that eating the same thing every day will provide the patient. For example, finding different flavors of the same snack bar or trying different types of snack bars can increase flexibility and prevent safety behaviors.

Sharing Calorie Counts with Patients

In addition to providing some of the same meals for convenience, we have found that some parents have found calorie counting to be an efficient way to navigate meal planning and meet their child's needs. We have experienced cases where parents and providers are unsure if the calorie expectations should be explained to their child. This is an important question as the comorbid OCD patients will have a higher susceptibility for rigidity and obsessionality. Sometimes when patients are aware of the calorie goal, especially those with comorbid OCD, they become so rigid that they have difficulty going even one calorie over (or sometimes one calorie under). At other times, the patient hay have been counting and obsessing over calories at all times throughout their ED. These patients often try to guess how many calories they are eating and regularly overestimate the calories in their meals. Alternatively, there are some patients who have been in recovery for a while but who still check calories obsessively as a compulsion related to their fear of relapsing or not doing the right thing in treatment.

We suggest that each case be looked at closely and that the decision to share or withhold calorie information be based on what fits best with the individual's fears. For patients who are having a difficult time tolerating anxiety around relapsing and are engaging in checking calories (in order to eat enough), we would suggest that they do not check and that calories are not discussed with them so they can gain tolerance for the idea that they may not have eaten enough. For patients who already know the calorie goal and are experiencing fear and rigidity around it, clinicians should work with parents to practice providing the patient with a meal that goes even 5–10 calories over what they are comfortable with to increase flexibility and DT. Alternatively, it may be best for some patients to not know their calorie goals at all or what is in their food to practice tolerating the overall uncertainty of caloric intake and to reduce any kind of negotiation at meals.

Providing Reassurance and Distraction

During FBT, parents are given a more autonomous role in feeding and weight restoration. Therapists act as expert consultants, empowering the parents to make most food decisions and encouraging them to find ways to successfully get their child to eat. Parents are also taught to distinguish their child's illness from their identity, which can help increase success by reducing the risk of criticism, blame, shame, hostility, or loss of temper. While trying different methods to get their child to eat, it is common for parents to say almost anything in desperation, such as "This is only two pieces of bread with some cheese, it won't affect your body." For most patients without OCD, this desperation comment may increase the likelihood of eating and, as long as it avoids criticism from parents, it may be beneficial for this goal (albeit possibly sending the wrong message about weight gain). If the child eats and becomes less malnourished, they may become more rational and reasonable about food, leading to further success and eventually recovery. However, for patients with OCD or obsessional thinking, this may not be the case. The child may have learned to eat based on reassurance and mental rituals, which may persist even with weight gain. This could explain why completing FBT, even with weight gain, may not always lead to the same recovery outcomes for patients with OCD comorbidity.

To improve outcomes for patients with OCD, we provide education about the disorder to the parents while using FBT. Previous research (Becker et al., 2020; Steinglass et al., 2011; Waller, 2016) suggests that AN is similar to an anxiety disorder, and that ERP may be an effective treatment approach. FBT may also be effective because it provides family-assisted ERP (Hildebrant et al., 2012). However, therapists who use FBT may not always be familiar with ERP, leading to poorly executed treatment from an exposure-based perspective. It is important for providers to understand the principles of exposure and be proficient in ERP to help families identify and eliminate safety behaviors that may interfere with progress. For example, allowing distractions while eating during FBT may inhibit the power of exposure and habituation, and remove the opportunity to practice DT.

In the early stages of treatment, it may be necessary for parents to provide verbal reassurance and distraction to get their child to eat more or to achieve initial weight gain (about 2.4 kg after the first month). This can help alleviate the psychological and physiological effects of AN and increase the parents' self-efficacy. However, once these goals have been achieved, it is important for parents to use language that is not reassuring and to provide opportunities for the child to sit with their anxiety related to the meal without distraction. For example, instead of saying "one meal won't make a big difference" or "it's okay, it's just whole grain toast," parents can try statements like "this is what we need to do so you can be strong enough for your sport" or "I'm sorry I have to do this, but regardless of what this food does to your body, it is what we need to do for your health." This can help prevent safety behaviors and ultimately strengthen treatment. Additionally, it may be helpful for parents to sometimes agree that the food may cause weight gain and encourage the patient to tolerate uncertainty.

OCD Activated by Loss of Control

Unlike other ED models, the patient is not voluntarily agreeing to treatment during FBT. As Chapter 9 pointed out, this involuntary handover of control around their diet, exercise, and social plans or sports can lead to heightened anger, sadness, and anxiety in many cases. When someone with OCD is confronted with unpleasant emotions or a stressful situation, symptoms can become activated. Additionally, as stated in Chapters 5 and 11, exposure is less successful when it is not volitional. Patients with OCD often engage in mental rituals and safety behaviors when anxious, and someone experiencing high levels of stress may have increased obsessionality and compulsions to escape unwanted exposures, reducing the effectiveness of treatment. This dynamic is not present in CBT-ED, as patients are collaborating and agreeing to treatment. However, individuals with significant AN are unlikely to agree to the necessary components of treatment in CBT-ED, so parents may need to act as temporary agents of change. At the same time, patients experiencing unwanted treatment may engage in surreptitious safety behaviors and may have increased flaring of OCD, hindering treatment.

To address the challenges faced by patients with both OCD and an ED, we recommend incorporating DBT principles (i.e., DT module) into treatment for patients. In addition, training parents to provide more elements of ERP into FBT may be beneficial. This is because children and adolescents with both conditions often experience high levels of distress, which can lead to increased OCD symptoms. By providing these patients with alternative ways to manage their distress, we can help reduce the stress of participating in FBT. Training parents in DBT skills, such as noncritical stance and emotion regulation, can also be helpful. This can enable them to practice these skills themselves and remind their children to use them when they are experiencing distress or rigidity. This may help reduce the activation of OCD in the early stages of the refeeding process. Overall, incorporating DBT principles and training parents in ERP techniques can be crucial in helping patients with OCD and an ED successfully participate in FBT.

Second, to improve treatment outcomes we suggest reevaluating how parents manage control over food during FBT. Currently, parents are responsible for making all food decisions and preparations during phase 1. However, we propose that the stress of this complete lack of control may increase OCD symptoms overall, and specifically the risk of patients using mental rituals to avoid exposure. To address these issues, we recommend training parents to incorporate elements of ERP that are missing from FBT, such as allowing patients to choose some foods (i.e., selecting between two options) within a hierarchy to increase volition. It is important that parents do not give in to the requests of the ED and choose foods that are more comfortable and accompanied by safety behaviors. For example, parents can offer the patient 2–3 relatively calorie-dense options and allow them to choose, with the understanding that the unselected options will be included in future meals. This not only gives the patient some control without sacrificing calories, it also eliminates a common safety behavior seen in FBT, whereby the child or adolescent feels anxiety or guilt during or after the meal and copes by reminding themselves that they were not the one who chose the meal to reduce their anxiety.

Adult Care

Chapter 2 reviewed the evidence-based treatment options for adults with AN. Although no single treatment has been identified as superior for this population, CBT-E has been the leading choice due to its transdiagnostic nature and some evidence of success in increasing weight gain. As mentioned in the section on BN and BED, CBT-E includes aspects of meal planning and exposure to specific foods. This section also highlighted how, for patients with a comorbidity of OCD, guidelines such as eating every four hours can encourage rigidity, which may be overlooked by clinicians who are not trained in ERP. In the case of adult AN specifically, the intense fear of weight gain can lead patients to report more distress around food and weight gain, as well as prompting more intense urges to use safety behaviors. We have observed that clinicians who are not trained in ERP may make mistakes that contribute to the weakening of treatment for this comorbidity.

Providing Reassurance and Distraction

Similar to how parents in FBT will often try anything to get their children to eat, clinicians may also say anything they can to encourage their adult patients to eat. It is common for clinicians to use reassurance to try to convince their patients to increase their intake or to incorporate more feared foods into their diets. This can present as a form of negotiation, with the therapist desperately trying to get the patient to agree. For example, a clinician may say to their patient "one slice of pizza won't cause any weight gain!" Clinicians who have a background in OCD treatment or who are familiar with ERP may be more aware of the need to encourage patients while also fostering their tolerance of uncertainty. When instructing patients in meal planning, it is important to avoid providing reassurance, as it can be used as a safety behavior by the patient. A stronger outcome may ensue if the patient cannot use the clinician's guidance as a safety behavior and has to tolerate the uncertainty of the outcome of eating the pizza (e.g., "I can eat this because they told me to"). Additionally, sometimes CBT-E recommends using distraction when the patient is having a hard time eating. This intervention should be monitored carefully for patients with a comorbidity of OCD, as the urge to use distraction and safety behaviors may not diminish as easily with weight gain in these patients compared to those without an OCD comorbidity.

Meal Planning Safety Behaviors

Many patients with AN have inflexible food and meal planning habits, especially those with a comorbidity of OCD. These patients may become accustomed to certain foods and rely on them for comfort and convenience, even if this limited diet is not nutritionally balanced. At first, this may not be a concern because weight gain is a priority in treatment, but it is important for clinicians to address this issue and encourage more flexibility in food choices as treatment progresses. Additionally, people with OCD may struggle to maintain flexibility in their food choices because they are prone to getting stuck on certain thoughts or behaviors. For example, Kaitlin (see Chapter 11) had a spontaneous recovery of her restaurant fears after quarantining during the pandemic. This highlights the importance of continuing to keep up on exposures posttreatment because with even accidental avoidance, especially with an OCD comorbidity, obsessions and fears can be very "sticky."

Additionally, even when patients are able to eat foods that they previously feared, they may still be engaging in safety behaviors. Vin, an adult patient with AN and OCD, had overcome his fear of cooking with oil and was able to prepare meals using olive oil. However, during a therapy session, it was revealed that he would only use exactly two tablespoons of oil and couldn't pour the oil straight from the bottle without measuring. This rigidity and safety behavior would not have been identified without asking specific questions about Vin's meal preparation habits. It is important to thoroughly question patients about their eating habits and behaviors in order to catch any issues that could hinder their recovery or increase the risk of relapse. Educating patients about safety behaviors can also be helpful, as they may be more likely to disclose these behaviors to you if you are unable to identify them during a session. Please see the following vignettes for more examples of safety behaviors used in meal planning and preparation.

Lauren

Lauren received CBT-ED for her AN as well as ERP for her OCD. During her ERP she realized and disclosed that although her food choices were adequate and her anxiety was much lower around food and weight gain, she discovered that she had been using a safety behavior in her meal planning. Lauren felt the need to put food on her plate in a way that looked "pretty, orderly," and overall "aesthetically pleasing." In explaining this behavior, she explained that almost every meal she ate at home needed to look like it could be "a social media post." Lauren felt some disgust when her plate of food looked less appealing, and the "pretty" aspect of the food allowed her to justify eating it. The aesthetic aspect of the food thus served as a safety behavior by suggesting that the food was "worthy" of being eaten. Lauren agreed to mess up her plate of food and eventually agreed to smashing her food before eating so it looked less appealing in order to counter this safety behavior.

Mary

Mary began CBT-E for AN and ERP for OCD. She had been avoiding a number of foods, including sandwiches. In treatment, she eventually agreed to eat sandwiches and planned to eat them during lunch. Eventually, Mary explained that she had been eating her sandwiches open-faced instead of together, citing that when she put the sandwich together "it felt like more calories." Mary was able to acknowledge that this line of thinking was not rooted in fact, and that it was influenced by her OCD-related magical thinking. Mary and her clinician had to be careful about addressing magical beliefs about food and safety behaviors, despite the general success of Mary eating more sandwiches.

Jamie

Jamie and his clinician were reviewing his progress during CBT-E for AN and adjusting treatment to address his health-related OCD. Although Jamie met the full criteria for AN, he also had a long history of health-based obsessions that sometimes affected his eating. Jamie noted that despite his successes with his food hierarchy in CBT-E, he realized that he would mentally review each challenge to feel better about his choice. For example, despite challenging himself to eat a candy bar for a snack instead of a "healthier" granola bar, Jamie would choose a Snickers bar and tell himself "well, this candy bar has peanuts in it, which is a healthy form of unsaturated fat." Jamie also became more comfortable eating pizza, but noted that he always added mushrooms or peppers to the pizza because "at least the vegetables are doing something for me." After identifying these safety behaviors, Jamie and his clinician set up exposures targeting stimuli that tapped into both his fear of weight gain and his intrusive thoughts about health.

In Summary

This chapter discusses the complexities of using meal planning interventions in the treatment of comorbid EDs and OCD. Evidence-based therapies for EDs often include guidance on meal planning, as disordered eating habits or starvation are central to the pathology of EDs. However, OCD can complicate ED treatment or be exacerbated by it. Clinical features of OCD, such as rigidity, perfectionism, intolerance of uncertainty, and seeking reassurance, can disrupt typical ED interventions such as meal planning. This chapter provides suggestions for addressing these complications in the use of meal planning in the treatment of comorbid EDs and OCD.

Navigating Self-Monitoring

As many clinicians already know, self-monitoring (in some capacity) is a core ingredient of virtually all CBTs. This is arguably *the* ingredient that helps patients really transition into being their own therapists, as this is where they learn to gather so much data about themselves. Self-monitoring enables people to play detective in their lives by learning how to detect their triggers, thought patterns, productive and unproductive behaviors, and moments of strength. This can be especially useful for EDs and OCD because the cognitions aligned with the pathology can feel so ego-syntonic and thus "sneaky" in that the afflicted person often has trouble discerning between their own thoughts and those of the pathology. Clinicians will often help patients better discern between the two by personifying or externalizing the pathology (e.g., "OCD said...," "My ED wants...," etc.). This enables the person to identify when they are experiencing thoughts that are produced by their illness. Although protocols such as CBT-E and ERP have a systematic layout in the treatment protocol where self-monitoring is introduced, the strategy of personifying the illness is somewhat related to self-monitoring and can technically be utilized before or after formal self-monitoring occurs. Before engaging in any type of formal CBT, many patients will come to treatment having already adopted the strategy of externalizing their illness. This can certainly be helpful to the treatment process, especially as it relates to compliance with self-monitoring.

As much of this book indicates, there can be many complicating variables that impact treatment when a co-occurring disorder of OCD is present. In the case of self-monitoring, however, the most notable concern is the potential for it to become compulsive. As clinicians who have treated OCD know all too well, any otherwise helpful skill or useful technique in treatment is fair game to become compulsive. Thus, clinicians doing ED treatment who may recommend self-monitoring ought to be aware of signs that OCD might be "ruining" it. When this happens, the value of self-monitoring can be completely overshadowed and the whole task can become part of OCD.

One of the most obvious signs of self-monitoring being "ruined" by OCD is level of distress. It is not necessarily uncommon for self-monitoring to evoke some degree of distress in patients with EDs because it inherently requires one to face the reality of their disordered eating, whether that be gravely undereating, subjectively overeating, objectively overeating, or binge eating. This can cause an uptick in distress for patients who prefer to stay as mindless as possible in their eating (e.g., "I just power through eating because I know I have to, I don't like to think about it or focus on it."). There is also an increased focus on food that comes with any type of food monitoring even in non-ED people. For individuals with EDs, this increased focus on food typically brings about distress. In fact, it is wise (and aligned with the CBT-E manual) to inform patients of the expected distress due to the heightened focus on food at the initial stage of self-monitoring. What is important to emphasize here is that the distress experienced in stand-alone EDs is expected to be short term, meaning that most patients habituate to this process after about two weeks of consistent monitoring. At this point in treatment, self-monitoring often becomes generally neutral or sometimes a nuisance, but it is rarely reported to be a continued source of distress. In the case of co-occurring OCD, however, habituation may not occur. Instead, the effect could be quite the contrary. One of the primary functions of self-monitoring is to provide us with more information. More information, especially measurable information that involves planning and scheduling wherein certainty and absolutes can be achieved (or seem as if they can be achieved) often fuels OCD. This is when self-monitoring related to food can become a problem.

When OCD is fueled, self-monitoring can activate prolonged distress, rigidity, and some degree of mindlessness because the person may be so fixated on doing it "exactly right" that they are not necessarily monitoring mindfully. This is problematic because another function of self-monitoring is to bring awareness and mindfulness into the eating setting. In this scenario, a clinician may see self-monitoring records that have very precise details about food with little to no thoughts, feelings, or comments. This is always something notable for clinicians to bring up in session.

As noted in Chapter 16 on meal planning, another tell that the monitoring has become compulsive is when the timing of eating and/or the foods consumed is exactly the same even after several weeks. It is important to note that patients are usually told that eating whatever they want, even if it is repetitive, is permissible in the beginning of ED treatment. It is generally expected that more flexibility in the timing and foods selected will occur as the patient moves through treatment and gets more used to the idea of a regular eating schedule. If, after several weeks of monitoring, you are finding this degree of specificity in the content of what your patients are reporting, it would be wise to neutrally inquire and to suggest switching things up a bit. If they are amenable to that with relatively little resistance, then perhaps OCD has "not attached itself" to self-monitoring. If there is an expression of agreeableness paired with difficulty for execution in real time, it is possible that OCD might have been activated. A desired exposure in this case would be to intentionally "mess up" the schedule.

Evaluating Problematic Patterns

When a clinician notices what seem to be possible compulsions on the self-monitoring record, it is helpful to bring it up in an unassuming fashion. For example, a patient may not verbalize in session "I am very rigid with my meal plan, so much so that I fixate on getting in every food group at every meal," but their self-monitoring records may end up being what reveals this problematic pattern. An example of this could be seen on a record "wonton soup, chicken fried rice, and vanilla yogurt." While there is nothing inherently problematic about eating vanilla yogurt with Chinese cuisine, it is certainly not typical or considered to be "normal." It is, however, how a person may approach meals when they have a compulsive need to plan meals "perfectly." In this scenario it may not even occur to the person that it is abnormal to combine these foods because of their fixation on following the guideline of having a food from each food group present at all meals, which is why they may not verbally report it. Thus, a clinician could gently point this out and inquire about the rationale for including yogurt with their dinner when reviewing the self-monitoring logs in session. It is possible that the rigidity would occur in the absence of monitoring and is more centered around the idea of "the perfect eating day," but it is our hunch that the written evidence of it only fuels OCD further. This could open the door to a useful exposure: messing up the self-monitoring log! This idea of "messing it up" could mean purposefully skipping days of monitoring, doing incomplete logs, falsifying the logs with incorrect reporting of food or eating times, or being dishonest in the reported thoughts and feelings section of the record (sometimes referred to as the context and comments). Ideally, the person would "mess up" both the record and the actual rigid eating pattern.

Another way that OCD can present on self-monitoring logs is in a compulsive need to overexplain or justify food decisions on the record. This behavior could be to reassure oneself about said food decisions and/or to avoid judgment from the therapist who will see the logs. This is particularly relevant for individuals who have obsessive beliefs in the morality category related to indulgence and gluttony, as mentioned in some of the cases in previous chapters. One case in Chapter 16 discussed "Jamie," who would overexplain his decision to eat a dessert. For example, he would often write down the nutritional breakdown of a Snickers bar in order to justify his decision to eat it. The peanuts within the bar would be labeled as a "healthy fat" on his self-monitoring record, which would decrease distress. This pattern prevented him from fully leaning into the experience of eating a dessert. He has a belief that eating a dessert just because it tastes good is gluttonous, which triggers obsessional thinking about his own morality. In this case it would make sense for his therapist to not only encourage ritual prevention about the over-explaining, but also to do exposure to eating other foods that have little to no nutritional value but taste good. This could even lead into an imaginal exposure about his gluttony evolving into other domains of immorality, enabling him to mentally expose to his core fear.

Calorie counting is another problem that may present in self-monitoring, whether purposefully or unintentionally. This problem is of course not exclusive to the ED-OCD overlap and occurs often in stand-alone EDs, but those with co-occurring OCD may have a harder time letting go of calorie counting. A self-monitoring record, while not focused on calorie counting, may serve to facilitate this problematic pattern. This problem was demonstrated in the case of Amanda (see Chapter 15), wherein her calorie counting became more a manifestation of OCD than of her AN. If calorie counting continues to be a problem after discussion about ways to prevent it, it may be advisable to have the person stop monitoring altogether to fully lean into the uncertainty about her intake. In Amanda's case, she noticed that when she stopped officially self-monitoring she continued to mentally note the calories in foods eaten throughout the day. However, she was unable to completely gauge her total for the day, or to even fully remember everything she had eaten, because she would sometimes do handfuls of X food here and handfuls of Y food later. This ended up being very valuable for her goals because uncertainty about her daily total was what took up most of her mental energy.

In Summary

As stated in the beginning of this chapter, the most notable consideration with self-monitoring is the tendency for it to become compulsive in some way. We know that this can happen with virtually all behaviors when a person has OCD. Avoiding self-monitoring altogether would likely not be indicated as you would lose useful clinical data and opportunities for exposure. Much of the process to mitigate any potential problems with self-monitoring will depend on your patient's specific patterns. Upon conversation and collaboration, exposures ought to be tailored accordingly. Furthermore, having a thorough understanding of your patient's OCD presentation will make you better able to predict some of these pitfalls and sidestep them in advance by changing some of the monitoring procedures.

Navigating the Scale & weighing

As discussed in earlier chapters, the most effective treatments for EDs (excluding IPT) incorporate a weighing component. Both CBT-E and FBT – the treatments with the strongest evidence base – use collaborative weighing at the beginning of each session. The primary uses for this intervention, discussed in detail in Chapter 6 and summarized in Chapter 9, include:

- Using weighing as an exposure;
- Practicing DT;
- Modeling neutrality or decreasing the value of weight for the patient;
- Providing corrective information and correcting the distorted cognition about the relationship between weight and food.

However, weighing can be challenging for patients with comorbid OCD due to their higher tendency for rigidity and reassurance seeking, and a decreased tolerance for uncertainty. Interventions related to collaborative weighing, including having the patient see their weight, using weight graphs, providing psychoeducation about scale precision and weight gain, the therapist's reaction to the weight, and the goal of increasing weight for restrictive disorders, may be affected by the disorder. This chapter will provide examples of how collaborative weighing can be difficult for these patients and offer suggestions for overcoming these challenges.

Weight Graphs and Psychoeducation

Weight graphs can be a useful tool in CBT for EDs by providing visual feedback, identifying patterns and obstacles, and helping the patient and therapist track progress toward treatment goals. They can also be used to reality-test the patient's theories about weight and related topics (e.g., metabolism) and as part of a behavioral experiment. Many manualized treatments for EDs, such as FBT and CBT-E, use weight graphs, but this intervention can be challenging for patients with comorbid OCD. In these cases, the therapist may need to adapt the use of weight graphs to address the specific needs and concerns of the patient. This is illustrated in the following vignette.

Erin

Erin is a 25-year-old white woman who works as a physician assistant student. She is in treatment for AN and OCD. She is in stage 1 of CBT-E and is targeting regular eating, practicing self-monitoring, and engaging in collaborative weighing at the beginning of each session. Erin's therapist is documenting her weight on a graph and has 10 weights documented.

Erin gained about 10 pounds in the first two months of treatment but has wavered between 115 lbs and 117 lbs for the last four weeks. Erin's therapist has noted that despite the psychoeducation provided to Erin earlier in treatment and her extensive medical understanding about the body given her profession, Erin often reacts to weight fluctuations as if they are more extreme than they are. Erin's OCD consists of a lot of checking behavior, including checking to see if she has all of her belongings, that stoves are turned off, that hairdryers are unplugged, and rewriting academic notes and work reports which causes her to be late to events and incurs occupational consequences.

ERIN: I am freaking out because I feel like all I am doing is gaining in here every week even though some weeks I eat less.

THERAPIST: I'm sorry you are freaking out, Erin. I want to point out that we have about 12 weeks of weights documented on your weight graph and that for the last 4 weeks there has been a trend of consistency rather than an upwards one.

ERIN: I know, but I've been thinking nonstop about how I was 115 last week and I was 117 the week before and now I am at 116 and I feel like my weight keeps going up nonstop.

THERAPIST: That is an interesting perspective, especially because your weight graph illustrates that you have gained a total of 10 pounds in 12 weeks which puts you at less than a pound a week overall. So we actually do not have any weight gain trends over the last 4 weeks. This presents a different understanding of your weight trend than "my weight keeps going up." You can even see from the line that we are plotting that yours has been quite flat for the last 4 weeks, which is typically the amount of time we use to establish a trend.

ERIN: Well, I feel differently about that trend. If my weight is one pound higher than it was two weeks ago, it seems like I am gaining. I feel like one pound is huge.

THERAPIST: Erin, I want to gently remind you about the information we discussed earlier in treatment along with the information on some of the handouts I gave to you about weight and body. We never interpret a single reading, mostly because that interpretation cannot be accurate given unknown variables like hydration, menstruation, state of bowels, etc. Medically speaking, a pound difference is unlikely to actually equate to changes in body mass but to shifts in the body. Remember the body is about 60% water weight, which will fluctuate frequently.

ERIN: I know, I know. That does make me feel better. I knew that myself too even before you told me. It helps when I hear it but then I tend to just go right back to obsessing about it. The movement from 115 to 116 does feel like a big jump and then I think about all the reasons why that happened – ugh, my brain just feels like it's on a loop.

In Erin's case, despite psychoeducation and a consistent weight range on the scale, she is still fixated on small fluctuations in her weight. This may be due to her OCD diagnosis, as people with OCD tend to be more rigid and obsessed with numbers and providing a weight graph. Even a minimal fluctuation may reinforce this obsession. For patients with AN, obsessions about numbers are often related to the effects of AN and starvation, which typically decrease with weight gain. However, Erin's comorbid OCD may make her obsessions more persistent and resistant to typical interventions such as increased calories and weight, reality-testing, and psychoeducation. In this case, psychoeducation about scale fluctuations may be experienced more as reassurance than education, and may not be effective. Instead of trying to reassure Erin that small weight changes are normal, it may be more helpful to embrace the uncertainty of the possibility that a small weight change is "true" weight gain. This approach may make weight graphs, which are meant to provide corrective information and reality-testing, less meaningful for patients with comorbid OCD. It may be more effective to interact with ED patients with OCD comorbidity in a way that acknowledges and tolerates uncertainty around weight. Let's revisit Erin.

ERIN: I am freaking out because I feel like all I am doing is gaining in here every week even though some weeks I eat less.

THERAPIST: Okay, and if that is actually happening, what does that mean?

ERIN: Well I am obsessing over the fact that I have ruined my metabolism and therefore lost my ability to restrict. Then, I think well if I am unhappy about my weight and want to change, I can't if my metabolism is broken. Also, it makes me feel that if I'm gaining weight on the weeks I restrict, when I actually eat what you've encouraged me to eat, I will literally gain 10 pounds in a week.

THERAPIST: Wow, it seems like your brain is having a lot of thoughts. Why don't we focus on the first fear, which sounds like you are worried you won't be able to handle bad body image days or you will be disappointed that you cannot change your body if you want to?

ERIN: Okay.

THERAPIST: Let's say that does happen and you have a day where you want to lose weight but are unable to. I'm wondering if you and I can talk more about tolerating bad feelings instead of jumping to fix the issue you have concern with. We may also want to practice learning to radically accept uncomfortable information.

ERIN: Yeah, I would rather lose weight than learn to deal but sure if I can no longer lose weight, I guess I would be open to that option.

THERAPIST: The second fear you are stating is that you are worried about your metabolism and believe if you eat 3 meals and three snacks a day as prescribed, you will gain 10 pounds in a week. I think that sounds like a theory we should test out. I know that you feel very uncomfortable about that idea but even if you did gain 10 pounds, that would meet your weight goal that you had agreed to as your healthy weight. Let's try to lean into that as a possibility this week and test out your hypothesis that your metabolism is so broken that when you eat 3 meals and 3 snacks, you will gain 10 pounds.

In this vignette with Erin, the therapist skipped the psychoeducation and the weight graph information and instead asked the patient to lean into her fears. The therapist suggested working toward tolerating the discomfort instead of using a behavior to feel better (i.e., restriction) and did not provide any psychoeducation to reassure the patient about her metabolism. Similarly, the therapist suggested the idea of gaining 10 pounds in a week as a positive outcome and framed the fear as an experiment without providing any reassurance about the likelihood of said outcome.

Jen

Jen, a 27-year-old teacher and soccer player with BN and OCD, illustrates how OCD can impact collaborative weighing. During therapy sessions, Jen always has to use the bathroom before being weighed and becomes fixated on the time of day, her watch, and the jewelry she is wearing. She also has rigid rituals around weighing herself at home, such as weighing herself naked at exactly 7am on a specific tile in her bathroom. Despite understanding that normal weight fluctuations and weight gain are not treatment goals and that the exact number is not important for therapy, Jen still wants to know her "exact weight." To address this, Jen's therapist suggests targeting avoidance of uncertainty and challenges Jen to stop engaging in her rituals. They also change the therapy times to challenge Jen's fear, as she finds night appointments particularly scary. The therapist also asks Jen to hold different objects while on the scale to tolerate not knowing her exact weight and to tolerate the possibility of the weight being higher without knowing how much is due to weight gain or the object she is holding. Her therapist also sometimes weaves in hidden weighing to further promote uncertainty about her weight.

Therapist Reactions

Therapists should be aware of their implicit biases and how they may influence their commentary and reality-testing during collaborative weighing with patients who have EDs and comorbid OCD. They should balance reality-testing and behavioral experiments with the understanding that weight gain itself is not necessarily negative, while also not reinforcing false beliefs about weight gain. It is important for therapists to avoid providing reassurance or safety behaviors to reduce the patient's anxiety during collaborative weighing, as this may reinforce false or negative beliefs or behaviors about weight gain and discomfort or anxiety. An example of a therapist providing reassurance about weight gain and reinforcing maintaining beliefs for their patient's anxiety is provided in the following dialogue:

THERAPIST: Hi Carl, nice to see you today. Let's start how we normally do and get your weight. Then we can process that experience and get to your self-monitoring records and any other agenda items we may need to get to.

CARL: Okay, sounds good. I really think I might gain weight this week because I was trying hard to achieve my goal of three meals. I know I haven't been able to add the snacks in yet but I did three meals a day almost every day this week when I only did it a couple times last week. I can tell I'm feeling resistant to seeing the number. I know I need to see it but I also have an exam for med school tomorrow and I am so afraid that this will screw up my night.

THERAPIST: That's great that you've been putting in such effort. I hear that you have a lot going on. It sounds like you may have in fact gained weight and you're worried it may ruin your day. I know you've been so anxious about your grades – if you don't want to get on this week, we could consider that because I don't want your day and studying to be ruined.

CARL: No, I know I need to. I always avoid and I need to learn how to stop avoiding everything.
Carl steps on scale and weight is up 1.5 pounds

CARL: Ugh. I knew it. I don't know if I can keep doing this. I feel like I'll weigh 1,000 pounds by the end of this treatment and I'll hate myself so much, I'll be so depressed. I am so upset because I know my anxiety is going to be so high today and I'm afraid I won't be able to concentrate.

THERAPIST: Hey Carl, I think it was really brave that you got on the scale and I hear that you are having a lot of anxiety and are worried your studying might not go as planned. I am also remembering that you told me since you stopped doing cardio exercise, that you've been lifting weights and doing more yoga. I'm wondering if it's possible that some of this weight gain is increased muscle mass?

CARL: Oh yeah, that could be true. I have been feeling stronger in my body. Maybe that weight gain was not from the three meals a day consistency and my change in exercise. I really like thinking this is muscle and not fat. I can't stand the thought of thinking my body has more fat on it. I think I'm going to think about that throughout the day so I'll be able to focus on my studies.

In this example, the clinician made a couple of errors that are potentially applicable to all ED patients, but especially to those with comorbid OCD. First, when considering the mechanisms of collaborative weighing, it is important to consider exposure, including habituation and inhibitory learning, as key factors for treatment success. Encouraging the patient to consider a thought that reduces their anxiety about the feared stimulus (e.g., gaining weight in muscle and not fat) undercuts the effectiveness of exposure. Instead, it is important to allow the patient to feel their anxiety during the exposure, attribute the weight gain to increased food intake, and learn to handle their anxiety without avoidance. Additionally, it is important to challenge the patient's beliefs about the relationship between anxiety and weight gain. In this case, the therapist discouraged them from weighing themselves and reinforced the patient's belief that anxiety would ruin their entire day. This type of reaction is not ideal for any ED patient, but is especially problematic for those with comorbid OCD. Almost all treatment for OCD involves removing safety behaviors, habituating to feared stimuli, and increasing one's ability to tolerate anxiety and other forms of distress. The therapist's response also reinforced the idea that being bigger is better if the weight is in muscle rather than fat, propagating weight stigma.

In cases wherein patients are resistant to weighing due to strong convictions or fear, MI may not be sufficient. In these situations, we have used certain interventions to help patients participate in traditional collaborative weighing. For example, we print out pictures of life-size scales with different readings and have the patient step on these pieces of paper in a hierarchical order. This allows for imaginal scale exposures and can help with self-efficacy and increase willingness to engage in the actual weighing process. Although it is an imaginal exposure, this intervention can still be framed as a behavioral experiment and help the patient test their beliefs ("even thinking about a higher number will ruin my day"). This gives opportunities to apply similar principles without actually stepping on the scale. However, it is important to communicate that eventually stepping on the scale is nonnegotiable for treatment. This conveys a few important messages: (1) that the patient can tolerate their anxiety, (2) that weight gain is not a bad thing, and (3) that the therapist believes in their ability to recover. By enriching this experience and communicating the principles of exposure, the therapist can help the patient experience anxiety without providing any safety behaviors or fatphobic responses, which can strengthen the effectiveness of this intervention.

Decrease in Weight as a Trigger

As mentioned in prior chapters, people with co-occurring EDs and OCD may become excessively concerned about the possibility of relapse. This fear may manifest in behaviors such as rigid meal planning or distress around changes in weight. For example, a patient with AN may have been accustomed to their clinicians expressing concern when they lose even just a couple pounds earlier in treatment when starvation effects were apparent. This internalized concern may not fade as treatment progresses, resulting in the patient feeling the same intensity after observing losing one pound when weight is restored as they did when they were underweight and malnourished. Similarly, a patient with BN who has an obsession around relapse may remember that not eating enough and lowered weights contributed to binge eating. As a result they now make sure to never let more than exactly four hours go by between meals and prefer rigidity regarding their weight. It is important for treatment providers to be aware of these issues and to work with patients to address their concerns and help them manage their OCD symptoms, as clinicians may inadvertently reinforce these fears due to their own investment in helping the patient achieve recovery and prevent relapse.

In cases where patients with EDs and OCD become excessively concerned about the possibility of relapse, at times it may be helpful to engage in hidden weighing. Although you may have gotten the impression up until now that seeing the weight is important in ED recovery, the suggestion for hidden weighing truly highlights the importance of understanding the factors maintaining your patient's disorder and then devising personalized interventions targeting those factors. By encouraging your patient to not see their weight, they are provided an opportunity to increase tolerance of uncertainty related to changes in weight. This intervention was utilized in the case of Jen, who was mentioned earlier in this chapter. The clinician should provide a rationale for this approach within the framework of ERP and expose the patient to statements such as "Maybe your weight is down this week and maybe you are close to relapsing." This may be difficult for the patient initially, but it can ultimately be beneficial for treatment in the long term. Further, it can be helpful to know the core fear of relapse (i.e., I'll miss out on senior year, I'll let my parents down, I am afraid of dying) and to identify and address compulsions (e.g., weighing themselves frequently to monitor weight) and reassurance seeking behaviors (e.g., mentally reviewing that they are lighter in the morning and therefore not at risk of relapse), and encourage the patient to abandon these behaviors. Instead, encourage your patient to face the possibility of relapse. This is important not only for managing OCD symptoms, but also when preparing the patient for the reality that setbacks and lapses in treatment can occur.

Hidden weights or similar interventions should be used after weight restoration for patients with restrictive disorders (i.e., ARFID, AN), and after a period of reduced binge eating for patients with BN and BED. The priority should be to help patients achieve physical health, and it may be dangerous for some patients to experience a decrease in weight earlier in treatment. This sequence of steps is consistent with the principles of ERP, which aims to expose patients to situations that are not objectively harmful. While it can be beneficial to occasionally remind patients that setbacks in treatment can serve a useful purpose (e.g., addressing missed triggers), it is important to do so infrequently or with caution, as this may be perceived as reassurance by the patient.

Some Helpful Points for Navigating Scale and Weight Exposures

- Personalized interventions should be devised to target the specific factors that maintain the patient's disorder.
- Knowing the core fear of relapse can be helpful in addressing underlying issues and providing the best course of treatment and directing weight exposures.
- Collaborative weighing is appropriate and needed for most patients.
    - Do not offer a hierarchy or an imaginal exposure without firmly encouraging in vivo weight exposures
    - A delay in collaborative weighing and scale exposure should be last resort
    - Have a rationale for why you are using a different technique
    - Balance a gentle but firm approach to help patients push through initial hesitation
    - Most people habituate to this exposure, including the therapist

- Most patients are not going to resist weight exposures
  - Many patients frequently weight check or, at the least, have a sense of what they weigh
  - Many patients will agree to weight exposures after receiving psychoeducation and rationale
- Be mindful that certain aspects of providing weight information (using weight graphs) can become obsessive with this comorbidity.
- Engaging in hidden weighing can be useful, and is helpful when the need is to increase tolerance of uncertainty related to changes in weight.
- Identify and address compulsions and escape behaviors, and encourage the patient to abandon these behaviors and face the possibility of relapse.
- This approach can be beneficial for treatment in the long term, preparing the patient for the reality that setbacks and lapses in treatment can occur.

In Summary

Weighing can be challenging for patients with ED and comorbid OCD due to their tendency toward rigidity, need for reassurance, and decreased tolerance for uncertainty. This chapter discussed the challenges that therapists may face when treating this comorbidity, including deciding when to use hidden or collaborative weighing interventions and when weight graphs may be less helpful. It also highlighted the importance of being aware of how psychoeducation about scale precision and weight gain, among other interventions, can become a safety behavior for these patients.

Navigating Body Image

Body image difficulties can be one of the most challenging aspects of treatment for clinicians, and tend to be a lasting source of pain for ED patients. Body image concerns can be a significant barrier to treatment success and may increase the risk of relapse (Shafran et al., 2004). Behaviors typically seen in ED presentations, such as body checking and scale avoidance, may be exacerbated when a patient has comorbid OCD

Body dissatisfaction and dysmorphia are common symptoms of EDs. They are often a result of a preoccupation with and overvaluation of the body, food, and the ability to control them, as well as starvation effects. However, body dissatisfaction is generally prevalent in the wider population due to a range of sociocultural factors. The media is highly implicated given the mass of misleading health advice along with different trends on social media (e.g., filters, diets) that can make people more anxious, aware, or insecure about their bodies (Tiggemann et al., 2017). Research has shown that the media plays a significant role in the development and maintenance of eating and shape-related disorders. Studies using various methods have all found that media has a strong impact. The internalization of societal pressures related to standards of attractiveness has been found to moderate or even mediate the media's impact on women's body satisfaction and ED risk (Thompson & Heinberg, 1999). Additionally, media and political environments often underrepresented and stereotype women, people of color (POC), and LGBTQIA+ individuals, perpetuating negative stereotypes and biases which have serious consequences related to the visibility and influence of these groups. This can further marginalize people and increase the focus on and impact of their appearance, which can lead to an intense association between worth and appearance (Barreto & Ellemers, 2005; Rudman & Phelan, 2008).

Given the widespread nature of body dissatisfaction and the influence of cultural messages that link a person's worth to appearance, it is not surprising that individuals with OCD may become more obsessive about these issues. This chapter will discuss how the interaction of OCD and EDs can uniquely present regarding body image, making treatment more challenging.

Body Checking and Avoidance

Body image related behaviors, such as checking and avoidance, are core symptoms of many ED presentations, but they are often intensified by comorbid OCD. These behaviors may include checking body parts with mirrors or avoiding mirrors altogether, inspecting body parts or avoiding looking at the body, trying on different sizes of clothing, comparing the current self to the previous self or others' bodies (often through pictures), or avoiding comparison altogether. Patients with comorbid OCD may have an intense presentation of these behaviors and a harder time discontinuing them due to their low DT, tendency toward rigidity, and proclivity for compulsive behaviors.

While these behaviors may sometimes resolve on their own as the patient eats more regularly, gains weight, or reduces other ED symptoms such as bingeing and purging, many patients (especially those with OCD) may need these behaviors to be targeted directly in treatment. While it is important for patients to feel comfortable and for the treatment environment to be conducive to successful eating, allowing the use of safety behaviors may undermine the usefulness of regular eating. For example, if a patient typically avoids eating large quantities or denser meals due to discomfort from fullness, wearing baggy pants during a large meal exposure may relieve that feeling and allow for easier eating. However, this may be an escape behavior and deprive the patient of the opportunity to practice DT. It is important for patients to succeed with eating early in treatment, but it is also important for them to become more accustomed to their bodies and to learn to tolerate discomfort from body changes such as weight gain or bloating after meals.

In CBT-ED (i.e., CBT-E and CBT-T), body image is addressed throughout treatment but is mostly targeted in the later stages (stage 3 of CBT-E and phase 5 of CBT-T, respectively). In FBT, it is not addressed at all. We recommend increasing psychoeducation and reducing safety or escape behaviors (such as wearing baggy clothes while eating ice cream) earlier on (after some weight restoration), especially in patients with comorbid OCD.

Kate

Kate, an 18-year-old patient with AN and a history of OCD, was in treatment during the summer before entering college. Kate and her mom were attending FBT sessions with the goal of gaining 20 pounds to return to her premorbid weight. Kate had a high level of avoidance and low tolerance for anxiety. After about 4 weeks of refeeding and gaining around 8 pounds, we instructed Kate's mom to devise exposures throughout the week that helped Kate eat in a way that increased her anxiety related to her body image and reduced safety behaviors.

Kate was more open to eating meals in private, but less so as regards eating on the beach where her family spent time during the summer. She would ask her mom to serve her meals at home so they could leave the beach for lunch and snack time, and then return to their friends and family. Although not engaging in manualized ERP, Kate's mom was provided with psychoeducation about the principles of ERP and family accommodation. Consequently, Kate was encouraged to eat her meals on the beach in her sundress, and eventually in just her bathing suit, where she had to tolerate the idea that others could possibly see her bloated stomach. This caused high levels of anxiety for Kate for several days until she reported that she no longer cared as much about this fear.

This use of an ERP technique related to body image, combined with refeeding, not only reduced Kate's anxiety around food but also helped to reduce the safety behaviors she had developed to make eating easier. Reducing avoidance behaviors because of body image concerns can also help reduce the emphasis on body image earlier in treatment, which may increase the likelihood that the patient will spend less time thinking about their body and reduce the overvaluation of it earlier in treatment. This can ultimately help to maintain recovery.

Body Image as an OCD Component

Body image dissatisfaction is a common symptom of EDs and is often exacerbated by comorbid OCD. Many people in Western culture have body image concerns and may become obsessed with their weight, along with their health, due to sociocultural influences. Fatphobia, along with the belief that body size is primarily a result of personal choices rather than genetics or biology, can contribute to negative stereotypes and negative emotions (i.e., disgust) toward individuals with higher weights. Individuals with OCD sometimes have preoccupations with morality and health concerns which can become entangled with body image in Western culture. The following sections outline some illustrations and suggestions for when this occurs.

Morality

People with morality-based OCD may become preoccupied with their weight as an embodiment of their fears about appearing indulgent, unvirtuous, or selfish. When an individual with OCD also has an ED (or subclinical eating behaviors), their body image concerns may be fueled by both their OCD and their desire for thinness. A patient with both an ED and OCD may have complex and intertwined body image concerns that need to be addressed in treatment. For example, some patients with morality-based OCD and an ED do not like to verbalize their concerns about body image for fear of seeming vapid and thus possibly being a bad person. Additionally, many of the patients with OCD mentioned in prior chapters (i.e., Margot, Kathy, Amanda) have strong fears around appearing gluttonous or overindulgent. Because society has (unfairly) tied higher weights to these characteristics, it makes sense that there might be a pursuit of thinness outside of an ED or exacerbation of already existing ED obsessions about thinness. Overall, because of harmful stereotypes associating body size and being virtuous, individuals with preoccupations of virtue and morality may be inclined to restrict their caloric intake or check their appearance in an effort to be seen as more virtuous.

Another aspect of OCD that can be associated with morality and body image relates to patients who may have internalized the societal message that they take up "too much space." This is particularly true for women, who from a young age often absorb messages about gender roles and expectations that can lead them to suppress their own needs, putting them at risk for depression and low self-worth (Elsesser, 2016; Jack, 1991). For example, one patient reported a fear of weight gain because she felt that taking up "extra" space was selfish. Another patient, who was higher in weight, experienced a tremendous amount of anxiety when flying because the airplane seats did not comfortably accommodate her body size. She felt guilty and thought she was making other people uncomfortable on the plane because she was "taking too much space" and being "selfish." To help these patients, approach this first with validation, support, and assistance in increasing their DT for these harmful ideas.

Health Fears

In addition to body image, another common misconception in society is that higher weights always lead to dangerous medical conditions such as cardiac issues and diabetes. Studies such as Flegal et al. (2013) indicate that weights associated with the lowest mortality are actually considered "overweight" (BMI 25–29.9 kg/m^2). In some cases, even those categorized "class I obesity" have a mortality advantage (Dixon et al., 2015). Similar findings have been reinforced by other research, such as Kvamme et al. (2012), which found an increase in mortality for those with a BMI below 25. Dixon et al. (2015) suggest that instead of prioritizing intentional weight loss, which may have uncertain outcomes for health, emphasis should be placed on promoting good nutrition, regular physical activity, fitness, and maintaining overall function in these weight ranges. However, this nuanced understanding of the relationship between weight and health is not widely disseminated via the media or health institutions. Despite medical research showing a more variable relationship between weight and health outcomes, many individuals still associate smaller bodies with good health and longevity, making those with OCD more susceptible to the pursuit of weight loss.

Many patients with intrusive thoughts about their health often fear conditions such as heart attacks, diabetes, and cancer. Due to the intense messaging linking higher weights (or obesity) with disease and doctors highlighting that larger bodies are risk factors for certain conditions (although correlation may not mean causation), many of these patients fear weight gain because they believe it will increase their likelihood of dying. For example, consider the case of Annie.

Annie

Annie, a 22-year-old nursing student with a severe history of AN, including multiple hospitalizations and moderate OCD (as measured by the YBOCS) is participating in CBT-E. Despite making significant progress, when Annie noticed her cholesterol was flagged on her lab results she became obsessed with cholesterol content, reverting back to checking labels and experiencing a spike in body image concerns. Her focus on weight gain was no longer driven by appearance concerns, but rather by a fear of having a heart attack later in life. However, in this case, the paradox is that cutting out foods, given her chronic AN, would likely cause her to relapse, bringing her closer to a heart attack. Through psychoeducation and ERP on her health concerns, Annie was able to resume normal CBT-E.

Annie's case not only highlights how health concerns can be associated with body image difficulties but underscores the importance of a functional analysis of symptoms and the accurate identification of the core fear for successful treatment.

Suggestions

Validation and Support

As clinicians, we must be careful to provide the right messages when responding to a fear of fatness or fears relating to the stigma for a higher weight individual. Providing support and validation is crucial. Given the intensity of fatphobia in Western society, along with its roots in racism and sexism (Stoll & Egner, 2021), clinicians should take care to acknowledge the potential for discrimination for those who have higher weights. Acknowledging where these messages come from and understanding the fear, while also not reinforcing that higher weights are inherently bad, is the balance one should find. Understanding the reality of these potential consequences while also providing tools to manage discrimination, including developing social support, problem-solving strategies, and DT, can enhance quality of life.

Psychoeducation

It is valuable to provide patients with the bank of knowledge that health outcomes are complicated and that body size or BMI in itself are typically not good markers of health or predictors of health issues later in life. Being mindful to not provide reassurance and ensuring there is communication with their physician to rule-out significant health risks can be helpful when treating patients with health fears.

Exposures

Reducing body checking may be hard for those with OCD. More intense measures (i.e., covering up mirrors at home) may be needed to disrupt rituals surrounding body image. Additionally, mirror exposure can be helpful for those who are avoiding their bodies or experiencing a lot of body dissatisfaction. There has been an increase in recent support for the use of mirror exposure alone or within the context of CBT with at least BN or BED patients (Trentowska et al., 2014). This may include standing in front of a full-length mirror, scanning the body or targeting a particular body part, and staring for about 20–30 minutes a day. Patients are to be aware of their levels of anxiety and monitor their thoughts, and may be encouraged to describe their body to themselves using neutral language. Practicing this along with other behaviors, such as going to stores and trying on clothes, and encouraging patients to wear tighter clothes, can assist in reducing maintaining behaviors.

Shifting Values

Chapter 6 emphasizes the significance of interpersonal effectiveness, shifting values, and increasing self-esteem as key mechanisms in the success of ED treatment. One effective way of achieving this is by placing more emphasis on other domains in a person's life, such as relationships, personal growth, and hobbies, which can help to reduce the importance placed on appearance and assist in overcoming body image struggles (Fairburn, 2008). Encouraging patients to engage in activities that they are passionate about can increase confidence and fulfillment, reducing the frequency and impact of negative thoughts about one's body. Pursuing interests and passions can also strengthen a sense of purpose and meaning in life, reducing the dependence on appearance as a source of validation and satisfaction. By increasing activity, social interaction, self-esteem, and diversifying one's identity (or not having all your eggs in one basket), a powerful force against body image issues can be created.

In Summary

Body image difficulties can be a significant challenge for clinicians treating ED patients, creating a barrier to treatment success and increasing the risk of relapse. Comorbid OCD can exacerbate ED behaviors such as body checking and scale avoidance. Body dissatisfaction and dysmorphia are common symptoms of EDs, but can also be prevalent in the general population due to sociocultural factors such as the media. Given the widespread nature of body dissatisfaction, it is not surprising that individuals with OCD may become more obsessive about these issues. It is therefore important for clinicians to be aware of how the interaction of OCD and EDs can uniquely present regarding body image given the associations between body and health or morality, making treatment more challenging. We recommend increasing psychoeducation and reducing safety or escape behaviors earlier on, especially in patients with comorbid OCD.

Part IV

Special Topics and Future Considerations

This section aims to highlight some of the additional variables that could further complicate the clinical presentation and corresponding treatment recommendations. Additionally, it discusses topics that are needed to best inform future research based on the current gaps in the literature and practice.

Special Topics and Challenges in Treatment

We would like to briefly highlight some of the additional variables that ought to be taken into consideration in treatment. Such variables have the potential to bolster or to thwart treatment. Not all variables mentioned in this chapter apply to all patients; they also can change over time and at different points in a patient's illness progression and treatment.

Severity of Illness

Severity of illness can impact how intensive the treatment needs to be (e.g., treatment approach, level of care, need for medical stabilization). A thorough assessment of severity is needed to prioritize symptoms (i.e., low pulse, orthostasis requiring hospitalization) (as highlighted in Chapters 14 and 15). Individuals with more severe presentations of EDs and OCD tend to have worse treatment outcomes overall (Garcia et al., 2010; Steinhousen, 2009), while those with mild to moderate presentations tend to have a quicker treatment response and a better prognosis (Herzog et al., 2022).

Chronicity of AN has also been linked to poorer outcomes (Scolnick et al., 2020). Patients with chronic EDs and OCD (stand-alone or co-occurring) may have less motivation for change (George et al., 2004) where their illness becomes entrenched with their identities. This is exemplified by the cases of Margot (Chapter 9) and Kathy (Chapter 13), who expressed difficulty imagining a life without their illnesses, which have become ingrained in their identities and daily decision-making. Social psychology indicates that low self-efficacy for change is linked to low motivation and goal abandonment (Margolis & McCabe 2006). This highlights the ebb and flow of motivation in patients presenting with ego-syntonic EDs and the need for motivational interviewing (MI). Perhaps more frequent contact (e.g., an email, text, brief phone call, or 30-min check in session) between weekly sessions could help to mitigate this pitfall. Since the severity of illness can vary over time and may fluctuate in response to stressors or other triggers, it is important to regularly assess the severity of an individual's symptoms and to adjust treatment accordingly.

Degree of Insight

Severity of illness, as well as a patient's perception of the illness severity, can affect the treatment process. Individuals with higher levels of insight into their OCD are more likely to stay in treatment and respond better to treatment, with better outcomes overall (Catapano et al., 2010; Steketee et al., 2011). Conversely, poor insight is associated with greater severity of symptoms, earlier age of onset, higher comorbidity for schizotypal personality disorder, poorer outcomes, more therapeutic trials, more frequent augmentation with antipsychotics, more treatment resistance, and lower willingness to make behavioral changes (Catapano et al., 2010).

Patients with high insight are more receptive to feedback and open to making changes to their thoughts and behaviors, which can facilitate the therapeutic process and help them develop healthier coping skills. To increase patient buy-in to treatment, clinicians should enhance their insight about the impact of their conditions through psychoeducation, MI, and feedback from others in their lives. This is especially important for patients with low insight before starting other treatment procedures.

Prior Treatment History

Patients having a prior treatment history can impact compliance and outcome in several ways. For reasons previously discussed, some patients have simply received bad treatment in the past. Bad treatment is arguably worse than no treatment at all because it leaves more for the new clinician to "undo" to optimize outcomes. This is rampant in ED treatment, where there are still many antiquated, nonempirically supported interventions being utilized in treatment centers all across the United States. For example, despite the most-studied and proven treatments indicating collaborative weighing as a vital ingredient to the protocol, many providers still choose to forgo in-session weighing altogether (or they engage in "hidden weighing"). This is a problem that many evidence-based ED providers encounter when working with patients with a prior treatment history. While some patients may quickly understand the rationale and agree to these interventions, clinicians should expect some degree of aversion or pushback from patients who find these behaviors to be "triggering" and who were previously accommodated by prior treatment providers. We often have to spend some additional time in sessions "unlearning" this avoidance. Let us briefly review a case to highlight this.

Allison

Allison is a 27-year-old female who has had OCD since childhood and an ED since early adolescence. She presented to treatment after having done a residential program, a partial hospitalization program, an intensive outpatient program, and years of weekly outpatient supportive talk therapy. In all treatments, providers either engaged in hidden weighing or avoided weighing completely (even at medical appointments), as well as ignoring her compulsive weighing due to her fear of others seeing her weight (despite compulsively weighing herself in private) and her high level of anxiety about weight gain. Her new clinician spent a lot of time on psychoeducation about how her current weighing habits served as maintenance variables to both the ED and OCD. This was followed by "selling" the rationale on collaborative in-session weighing and ritual prevention of at-home weighing. She was completely unwilling to budge on this at first, but with persistence, conviction, and collaboration from the new therapist, she was able to make gradual movement. The therapist did a gradual exposure and ritual prevention process.

The process involved reducing the frequency of weighing to once a day, then moving the scale to the therapist's office for a night, with the agreement that the patient could have the scale back at any time. Over time, the days with the scale at the office gradually increased. The exposure therapy also involved different levels of weight exposure, starting with the patient getting on the scale alone, then with the therapist in the room but not looking, and gradually increasing to a collaborative weighing where both the patient and therapist see the weight together. This continued over several sessions until the patient was collaborative weighing and was also able to weigh at medical appointments. The focus later shifted to the patient's OCD, and the ERP sessions had to incorporate collaborative weighing as an exposure even though her eating was no longer the focus of the treatment. The patient eventually overcame her fear of weighing.

As this case highlights, Allison had a lot of unlearning to do related to the scale and its use in health care appointments. This initial degree of unwillingness did not exclude her from treatment, but the clinician had to do some creative problem-solving to ensure that Allison agreed to work toward collaborative weighing. This process certainly prolonged treatment by delaying a vital ingredient to uproot her ED psychopathology.

In the world of OCD treatment, sometimes patients participate in general CBT treatment or supportive talk therapy that inadvertently provides reassurance or avoidance and can strengthen OCD over time. An example of this is the case of Billy.

Billy

Billy is a 33-year-old male who, since early childhood, has a history of OCD focused on being a "good" and moral person. Examples of his fears include the possibility of sexually molesting his niece and nephew, poisoning his dog with bleach or rubbing alcohol, undressing in public, etc., along with less distressing obsessions (i.e., doors unlocked, leaving lights on). Billy was quite compliant with ritual prevention (e.g., leaving the house without checking the lock at all). This weakened his obsessional thoughts about such content quite significantly. For the former set of obsessions, he was not as compliant with treatment recommendations both inside and outside of session. He would often engage in reassurance seeking behaviors of various forms and employed avoidance strategies (e.g., always having his mom present in the room when he played with his niece or nephew, never taking either of them to the bathroom to be changed, not keeping bleach in the house, etc.). While he stated that he understood the rationale for imaginal exposure in session, he was reluctant to engage in the process, citing the rationale "No normal person would want to think about themselves molesting a child or hurting their dog!" Billy also stated that this intervention seems "so far off from what I have done in prior treatment for OCD," despite the previous treatment having poor outcomes. Even upon showing Billy literature from other OCD specialists indicating that imaginal exposure to graphic images is standard protocol in ERP, he was reluctant. He began to miss appointments, claiming other obligations and scheduling conflicts, until he eventually reached out to terminate treatment. He was also unwilling to do a termination session to wrap up and discuss his reason for prematurely ending treatment; however, he did briefly indicate that he felt the prescribed treatment approach was not a good fit for his needs. This type of scenario is an unfortunate outcome in some rounds of exposure therapy, especially when the patient has been given other options before (regardless of their efficacy).

Billy's prior treatment history may have contributed to premature termination. Ways to sidestep this pitfall could include spending a fair amount of time (perhaps more than the manual would indicate) discussing the rationale, any concerns the patient may have prior to beginning treatment, and connecting them with others who have seen success with exposure therapy. Such conversations ought to include a lot of empathy and validation about the proposed changes and the degree of difficulty that comes with it. It is well documented that a strong alliance is a vital ingredient in all psychotherapies, lessening the likelihood of premature termination (Cournoyer et al., 2007).

Other miscellaneous issues that might come up due to a patient's prior treatment history relate to the therapeutic orientation and messaging surrounding hope.

Treatment Orientation

The importance of research-based, present-focused, behaviorally driven treatment plans targeting the variables that maintain psychopathology may not have been emphasized by all previous healthcare providers. Some providers may have focused on underlying issues such as trauma, family dynamics, self-esteem, body image, depression, and anxiety, rather than breaking problematic cycles in patients' lives. Empirically supported treatments, such as FBT, focus on breaking problematic cycles rather than exploring the underlying causes of illness. This difference in approach may be off-putting to patients and families who have been led to believe that improving body image or resolving past trauma will lead to recovery. It's important to have a conversation about this difference and the rationale behind it to ensure patient (and family) buy-in and willingness to proceed.

Degree of Hope

A person's perception of their illness and their level of hope for improvement is crucial to sustained motivation and a successful outcome in treatment. Having gone through multiple rounds of previous treatments can decrease hope for success, and past providers may have given negative messaging about the prognosis, especially in cases of chronic illness. This harmful messaging needs to be addressed and undone in order to set the patient up for success in this new round of treatment. The clinician should assess the past messaging and, if applicable, validate how it has been discouraging. Speaking with conviction about hope for change in this new treatment is crucial. This will likely improve the therapeutic alliance and improve treatment adherence, limit resistance, and decrease the likelihood of relapse by highlighting self-empowerment and autonomy. Failing to address this aspect of the patient's treatment history could miss an opportunity to dispel harmful beliefs about the helpfulness of treatment and the mental health system.

Religious and Cultural Variables

The religious and cultural background of a person should be taken into consideration when treating EDs and OCD. Stigma around mental health and treatment may exist in some cultures and religions. There may also be cultural and religious differences in views on treatment, such as preference for holistic or faith-based approaches over symptom-focused treatments. Additionally, some cultures and religions may disapprove of the use of psychotropic medications, so it is important to educate patients about potential benefits but also respect their autonomy if they choose not to take them. Clinicians should manage these variables in an ethical and culturally sensitive manner.

Clinicians must be aware of cultural and religious differences in beliefs about body shape, size, and food practices, as well as religious rituals such as fasting and prayer. For instance, a patient who follows Orthodox Judaism may have obsessions and compulsions related to their kosher diet and religious laws regarding opposite-sex contact and touch. In these cases, it is important not to assume that all religious beliefs are a result of pathology and to consult with a religious leader, such as a Rabbi, to determine which beliefs and rituals can and cannot be challenged in therapy. This demonstrates a commitment to respect the patient's cultural and religious identity and can strengthen the therapeutic alliance. It is also crucial to understand and respect cultural differences in beliefs and norms related to body weight and shape. Different cultures have varying ideals, and it is not the role of the clinician to criticize or judge them. Patients may find it difficult to give up weight control behaviors and beliefs that do not align with their culture's ideals. It is the clinician's job to support and guide them in accepting these differences, rather than trying to prove that their cultural ideals are incorrect. This applies to all cultural groups, including those within a particular community. Our focus should be on inquiring, educating, and respecting patient autonomy. We will briefly outline the case of Arden to highlight this.

Arden

Arden is a 15-year-old white female with a long history of food rigidity that later turned into AN. She is from a very affluent community where "healthy, clean" eating is the norm by virtually all of her peers and their families. Exercise and maintenance of a lean, athletic physique are also the community's norm. To put simply, disordered eating is quite normalized and sometimes even glorified in her affluent community. Already we can see how this may pose a bit of a problem for AN treatment both by way of getting Arden to gain weight in addition to helping her to let go of these beliefs about weight, food, and fitness.

In Arden's case, the goal of weight gain along with various food exposures remains nonnegotiable, but we may have to reconsider what recovery looks like for Arden within the context of her culture. For example, all of her friends and family (who do not have diagnosable EDs) primarily only eat cauliflower pasta and pizza crust instead of flour-based crust. Asking her to get fast food would be met with shock and unwillingness due to her community norms. We would encourage clinicians to navigate the differences between cultural norms and accommodation when picking and choosing battles during treatment planning. In Arden's case, she was successful in eating flour-based pasta and pizza crust; however, she expressed disinterest in consuming these foods regularly. Because many individuals have less than ideal habits around food in today's world, certain eating preferences, especially considering cultural/community norms, should be respected. Even if we believe that it is disordered to consume mostly cauliflower-based pasta or pizza, this would not necessarily preclude a patient from being considered recovered once they have completed treatment, are weight restored, and do not report much distress around food and body. Helping your patient achieve their goals in recovery while living a life that is not impairing or dysfunctional should be the primary targets. Clinicians should not push our beliefs, values, norms, or ideals on our patients if it is possible for them to reach symptom remission within the values and norms of their given culture.

Family and Social Support Variables

Families and social support are crucial for the treatment process, particularly for adolescent and young adult patients. It is important to note that a stable family and good social support are not essential for treatment success, but they can certainly help the process. When these supports are lacking or problematic, it can create additional challenges for the clinician and may require adjustments to the treatment plan as issues arise.

Accommodation

Family accommodation (briefly discussed in Chapter 3 and reviewed in Chapter 11) refers to the ways in which family members adjust their behaviors and routines in response to the symptoms of a loved one with OCD or an ED. This accommodation can have both positive and negative effects on treatment (Storch et al., 2007). Although support and relieving distress is the intent, it can also perpetuate the problem and make it harder for the patient to recover. For example, family members may engage in obsessional thinking, provide resources for compulsions, avoid feared stimuli, and provide excessive reassurance. It's important for clinicians to be aware of the role of family accommodation in the treatment of OCD and EDs and to work with families to address these issues. The case of Kathy (mentioned in Chapter 13) is a good example to highlight this.

Kathy's husband not only minimizes how severe her presentation is (possibly due to the distress he would experience by acknowledging how impaired his wife is), he also provides reassurance to her regularly about her eating, germs, and cleanliness, that she is a good person, that people like her, etc. The list can go on and on. He also makes many accommodations for her compulsions (i.e., providing more luggage to pack cleaning supplies and personal bedding, trying not to upset her). All this accommodation, while well-intended to preserve a sense of mental peace for both of them, has only exacerbated her symptoms over time. This example highlights how these illnesses worsen by "tricking" not only the person afflicted but their loved ones as well.

Other examples of accommodation include but are not exclusive to the following: parents continuing to buy all of their child's requested "safe foods," writing notes for requested extensions on school work due to time-inefficient compulsions, giving permission for their child to eat less than needed at a meal, paying for more services or appointments with providers to quell distress, advocating for hidden weighing, calling treatment centers to request changes to the usual programming, getting up early to allow their child to complete rituals before needing to leave the house, agreeing to find a new treatment provider if the selected one proposes exposure-based methods, etc. Family accommodation can reinforce compulsive behaviors, decrease motivation for treatment, and interfere with progress in treatment (Marien et al., 2009; Storch et al., 2007). It is important for clinicians to educate families on the negative impact of accommodation and work with them to address these issues.

Communication

Although the intention is usually not to be harmful or unsupportive, a lack of proper communication can lead to the person with ED or OCD feeling unsupported. Some families may have difficulty communicating effectively or resolving conflicts, which can lead to misunderstandings and perpetuate the pathology. Adolescents may have more difficulty staying engaged and motivated for change without adequate support from their family. Without proper communication, it is difficult to provide the necessary support. Additionally, high levels of criticism and anger from family members can be detrimental to recovery and have been linked to higher rates of relapse, as well as increased anxiety and depression posttreatment (Steketee, 1993). This is particularly relevant in FBT, wherein parents' ability to remain emotionally regulated when their child's symptoms are flaring up is crucial to a successful outcome (Allan et al., 2018).

Some families may not provide adequate support for their loved one due to a lack of understanding of the disorder, personal issues related to the disorder, or other conflicting priorities (i.e., losing a job, having another baby). If a support person is having their own issues related to the disorder, it is very important that clinicians be aware that their distress or bias can influence how well they support the treatment plan. A case example to highlight this problem is Brielle.

Brielle

Brielle is a 24-year-old white female who has had a co-occurring presentation of OCD and atypical AN since her late childhood/early adolescence. She comes from a family with tremendous financial privilege, wherein many accommodations have been made and could continue to be made due to their available resources. Brielle has spoken to her therapist at length about her mother's extreme relationship with exercise and restrictive eating, along with her frustration around her mother's denial of her own eating issues, going so far as to identify her mother as a primary trigger.

The combination of her family's financial privilege and her mother's relationship to food and exercise presented a barrier to treatment in a variety of ways. The first is that Brielle had never directly told her mother how her behaviors impacted her and her mother never acknowledged any problem in her own behaviors, describing it as a "lifestyle" that she was unwilling to change. Another way this served as problematic was that foods provided as exposures and homeworks were never in the house. When Brielle was in a residential treatment center, she would often call home to complain about the food served despite the food being normal (i.e., turkey and cheese sandwiches).

Reassurance, reinforcement of food myths, modeling unhealthy behavior, etc., were all significant obstacles for Brielle to overcome.

In Summary

The variables and examples mentioned throughout this chapter certainly do not preclude your patients from engaging in treatment, nor do they mean that a positive outcome is unlikely. However, clinicians ought to spend adequate time on assessment of these variables and intervene in a collaborative manner wherever possible. This may require you to think outside of the box to help individuals and families better access appropriate services, formulate and maintain hope, and develop better communication strategies and coping skills for distress in order to establish a supportive, collaborative treatment environment that will be conducive to a positive outcome.

Continued Research

As we end this book, we want to highlight some additional areas for research consideration and practice. It is important to note that there is still much to be understood in regards to treating the co-occurring presentation of OCD and EDs. While further examination is needed in the broader context of treatment, there are a few key areas that should be considered for best practice.

Special Populations

There are several special populations that may need additional considerations when approaching assessment and treatment planning.

Older Adults

Older adults have been somewhat left out of the mental health conversation until more recent years, likely due to underreporting and underutilization of services for mental health (Brody & Kleban, 1981). Older adults with OCD or EDs may have been living with their symptoms for many years due to lack of mental health resources or information in prior generations, resulting in internalized and accepted symptoms. Over time, these symptoms may become more ingrained and may not appear unusual to the individual. Due to this, it may not be immediately evident to them that their beliefs and behaviors need treatment, leading them to need more MI during treatment. Staying aware of their physical and cognitive presentation and health changes is important as it may impact their presentation and/or interfere with treatment. For example, older adults may be more mindful of foods with higher cholesterol or sodium and may have received recommendations from their doctor regarding their diet and exercise. Because having OCD and/or an ED can intensify a person's need to follow a recommendation "perfectly" or to an extreme, this population may be more at risk of obsessing over these topics. Lastly, older adults are often facing difficult experiences related to death and loss. They may have family and peers who have died, while possibly dealing with the idea of death for themselves or a loved one; thus, anxiety and fears about death may be commonplace. Depending on your patient's health, cognitive functioning, and pathology severity, it may be helpful to consult with a loved one, such as one of their adult children, or with their medical provider, if appropriate.

Pregnant and Postpartum Individuals

Pregnant and postpartum individuals present unique considerations within the context of OCD and EDs. Hormonal changes, stress, and altered sleep patterns can all impact mental health during this stage of life, which can vary greatly depending on social support and financial privilege. For individuals already struggling with OCD and EDs, their symptoms may reemerge or intensify during pregnancy and postpartum. Two important factors to note include changes in body shape and weight, and the fluidity of OCD symptoms. It is important for clinicians to be aware of these factors and to tailor their approach accordingly.

The average pregnant person gains approximately 25–45 pounds, depending on their prepregnancy weight (Rasmussen & Yaktine, 2009). Body changes during pregnancy, including changes in shape, skin structure, and general appearance, can pose challenges for individuals with pre-existing body image issues and EDs. Treatment plans may need to be adjusted to address these changes and their impact on mental health. For example, changes in diet, weight, and nutritional intake may lead to an increase in ED cognitions, and some individuals may continue to struggle with ED behaviors throughout pregnancy. Being weighed and possibly having to discuss weight changes is also a routine part of perinatal appointments that may activate symptoms. Clinicians should consider discussing these concerns with the obstetrician from the start of treatment if necessary. It is important to be mindful of these unique challenges and to tailor treatment accordingly. Likewise, it is

Regarding OCD in pregnant individuals, Clinicians ought to remind themselves that OCD can "attack" what a person cares about most in life, and for many individuals their future child or new baby falls into that category. This can result in excessive reassurance seeking behaviors and over-involvement in medical recommendations and information about pregnancy, birth, and infancy, which can increase anxiety and fuel OCD cognitions. Using tools such as a heartbeat Doppler, although not inherently problematic, can provide reassurance, but for individuals with OCD this could trigger compulsive behaviors. To avoid the reassurance-compulsion cycle, it may be recommended not to use a Doppler and instead to provide limited information to ease anxiety in individuals with OCD during pregnancy.

LGBTQIA+

The LGBTQIA+ community needs further research and resources related to their healthcare. While there have been improvements throughout recent years, there is still much about their health trajectories, presentations, and needs for treatment that is unknown and/or not available to many LGBTQIA+ individuals. The same is true when we consider their needs within OCD-ED treatment, especially when we take into account the discrimination, stigma, and general stressors that impact this population. Research has documented that those within the LGBTQIA+ community are particularly vulnerable to developing an ED and OCD (Gordon et al., 2021; McClain & Peebles, 2016). Body dysphoria and trauma may play a role in the development of these issues, where body image issues can also extend beyond EDs. For LGBTQIA+ individuals with OCD, there may be obsessions related to religious scrupulosity, morality, and contamination based on messages received from families, peers, and society. It is important for clinicians to differentiate between genuine internalized homophobia or transphobia and OCD, as the former is typically processed and managed differently from OCD.

Clinicians should allow for extra time in the assessment phase of treatment for LGBTQIA+ individuals and seek appropriate consultation as needed to provide a safe, supportive, and culturally competent environment.

Co-Occurring Conditions

Individuals with co-occurring conditions will naturally present to treatment with additional variables and needs to consider, as they may complicate treatment procedures and worsen outcomes. Common co-occurring conditions to both OCD and ED include the following: anxiety disorders, MDD, PTSD, autism, and personality disorders (Graber & Brooks-Gunn, 2001; Whitehead & Suveg, 2016; Cassin & von Ranson, 2005; Boger et al., 2020; Murray et al., 2015; Trottier & MacDonald, 2017; Pinto et al., 2011; Madowitz et al., 2015; Semiz et al., 2014).

The treatment for ED-OCD may need to be adapted based on other treatments the patient is receiving. For instance, if the patient is undergoing substance abuse rehabilitation or attending a DBT skills group, treatment for ED-OCD may need to be temporarily paused. It's important to keep in mind that many providers in other fields may not have a comprehensive understanding of EDs or OCD, so clinicians should communicate with other providers to ensure consistent messaging for the patient. To prevent mixed messaging, it may be helpful to have a brief conversation with other providers to explain the cycle of OCD and how ERP works.

Children

There are several considerations that clinicians ought to take into account when treating children with co-occurring OCD and EDs. Developmental stage is the first notable consideration. Clinicians should consider their comfort level in working with and using age-appropriate modified interventions (i.e., rephrasing psychoeducation, using shorter or more frequent sessions, using additional forms of positive reinforcement, e.g., a small prize or sticker). As stated in Chapter 20 under "accommodation," family involvement is highly influential for the efficacy of treatment for both EDs and OCD (Lock & Le Grange, 2005; Marien et al., 2009; Storch et al., 2007), especially with children. Forming a strong rapport that encourages active engagement from parents will be crucial to treatment success. Additionally, clinicians ought to have at least some contact with school personnel to communicate the treatment plan and discuss the child's needs while at school. For example, some exposures may need to occur in school, a child may need to have supervised lunches, etc. Overall, it is important for clinicians to be aware of the unique needs and challenges of working with children and tailor the treatment accordingly.

POC

When treating POC with OCD and EDs, clinicians must be aware of the added burden of discrimination and cultural factors that may affect the development and maintenance of these disorders. Factors such as the stress from discrimination may lead to maladaptive coping strategies and issues such as SUDs or EDs. Historically, the term "obesity" has been discriminatory to POC, particularly black bodies. Many argue that the flawed BMI scale, that was originally normed on white men, perpetuates racial, not scientific, expectations on how certain bodies should exist. Additionally, cortisol, which is associated with weight gain, is also associated with stress from discrimination (Carter et al., 2019). It is important to recognize that these disorders are not limited to a specific race or ethnicity and that the stereotype of them being a "white woman's problem" can lead to underdiagnosis and lack of understanding among POC. Clinicians should strive to create a safe and inclusive therapeutic environment and be aware of their own cultural biases. They should also take into consideration the cultural differences that may affect body image standards, food choices, and the definition of recovery even though the road to getting competent care can be difficult (Mikhail & Klump, 2021; Uri et al., 2021).

Clinicians should ask thorough questions and be open to discussing appearance-related concerns if there are differences of race, culture, and religion between the provider and patient. Additionally, POC with OCD may have obsessions related to race discrimination and safety that can not only present as intrusive or distressing, but which are reinforced by daily microaggressions. For example, a black man with OCD may have obsessions about getting pulled over by a police officer while driving. He may then engage in corresponding compulsions while on the road that not only impact his quality of life but also paradoxically increase his chances of getting pulled over. His anxiety may then be conveyed to the police officer, which could be misconstrued and have dangerous implications. This example highlights a concern that ought to be met with sensitivity and awareness to the actual risk for harm when living in the world as a POC.

Athletes

When treating athletes with OCD and EDs, clinicians should be aware of the unique stressors and pressures that they may face in relation to their sport and performance. Athletes may experience a great deal of pressure to maintain a certain weight or body composition, which can contribute to the development of disordered eating patterns and body image concerns. Additionally, athletes may be at risk for OCD due to the need for perfectionism and control in their sport, which can manifest as obsessive thoughts and behaviors. Gymnastics, for example, requires precision not only to be successful in the sport but also for safety reasons. Repetition to achieve perfection is therefore encouraged in the sport, and is arguably essential. If a gymnast is even slightly off with the placement of their foot on a 4 inch beam, their mechanics can shift leading to a poor landing. This will result in not only a lower score, but also could risk a dangerous injury (e.g., broken neck).

In treating athletes with ED-OCD, it's important to consider the impact of their sport on their recovery. Athletes may feel pressurized to return to competition before they are fully recovered, and may face difficulties managing the ritualized behaviors that are common in sports. Clinicians should be mindful of external pressures from coaches, parents, and peers and work with athletes and their teams to develop a treatment plan that balances their mental health and their ability to compete. This may involve modifying treatment to accommodate other services, such as substance rehabilitation or DBT skills groups, and avoiding mixed messaging from different mental health providers. It's also important to note that the exercise and diet requirements of the sport may conflict with ED or OCD treatment, so this should be taken into consideration when developing a plan.

Therapist Attitudes and Training

As discussed in Chapter 11, therapist attitudes about exposure therapy can have a significant impact on treatment outcomes for patients. Positive attitudes lead to more effective use of the therapy, while negative or neutral attitudes may lead to lower confidence and increased anxiety. There is a gap in clinician training for exposure-based methods, especially in rural areas, and the utilization of exposure therapy is often low. Further research is needed to examine the reasons for the underutilization of exposure therapy and ways to better disseminate it. The pandemic has shown that virtual platforms can be efficient and cost-effective for training, and further examination of clinician barriers for exposure therapy with ED treatment is warranted.

Possible Treatment Contraindications

Although the leading treatments (i.e., FBT, CBT-E, ERP) for the individual disorders of this comorbidity are robust and demonstrate strong outcomes in the literature, data still suggests that not everyone reaches remission and that there are some moderators for treatment outcomes. More research needs to be done to identify these variables and provide adaptations to improve outcomes for certain subgroups. To underscore messaging from prior chapters, we know that EDs have a high risk for medical complications (Bulik et al., 2021; Miller et al., 2005) and suicidal ideation (Papadopoulos, 2009). Any acute concern for either would warrant immediate attention and supersede other symptoms and treatment plan goals. After stabilization and ensuring safety, patients can resume their course of ED-OCD treatment.

FBT

There are some possible contraindications to discuss.

Parental Factors

It has been suggested that even low levels of parental criticism have a negative impact on FBT outcomes (Allen et al., 2018; Loeb & LeGrange, 2009). Given this, one could assume that abuse toward the child is contraindicated. Abuse in the home poses a risk not only as a deterrent to ED treatment, but also in terms of threatening the overall well-being and safety of the child. ED specialists should be familiar with local child protective services (CPS) and collaborate with them when addressing suspected or disclosed child maltreatment in patients undergoing FBT. If working with a caregiver raises safety concerns or if CPS professionals indicate caregiver involvement is not possible, alternatives such as involving other family members or individual therapy can be discussed with CPS (Kimber et al., 2020). For more on this topic, please see the studies by Kimber et al. (2019) and Kimber at al. (2020).

Families who do not fit the traditional Western two-parent family norm may need additional FBT sessions to achieve similar remission rates (Lock et al., 2005). Additionally, clinicians should caution against using FBT in cases wherein there is an acrimonious divorce with shared custody. It is very important in FBT that parents present a unified front against their child's ED. Plenty of divorced parents coparent well, and while flawless coparenting is not essential, there needs to be a basic understanding from all parties that external marital and financial discord must be tabled throughout the proceedings of FBT.

OCD

Lock and Le Grange (2019) noted that those with co-occurring OCD tend to fare worse in FBT compared to peers without OCD. We have also noted this in clinical practice. We have not only seen that co-occurring OCD worsens outcomes in FBT, we have also seen that FBT can worsen OCD symptoms. We expanded upon this in further detail in Chapter 9. However, we want to make clear that such observations are merely anecdotal, and thus we are not implying that a co-occurring diagnosis of OCD precludes one from engaging in FBT or from successfully completing it. We are simply suggesting, consistent with the messaging provided by Lock and Le Grange (2019), that modifications may be needed (as mentioned in Chapter 16). Furthermore, we think that it would be informative and helpful for this observation to be examined empirically.

Motivation and Goals

The last two points to mention regarding contraindications relate to the very nature of all CBTs, including exposure-based interventions. Collaboration is a core component of all CBTs. Therefore, we need to have some degree of patient motivation and volition for the proposed interventions for the alliance to remain strong and for the treatment to be effective. Overall, patients need to understand the rationale for interventions and have a general commitment to reach the goals set at the beginning of treatment. We would advise clinicians to not move forward with CBT-based interventions if patients are still disinterested in the goals after proper MI and psychoeducation occur. Furthermore, we advise clinicians to explain to patients why a discontinuation of treatment at the current time is better for them in the long-term rather than "forcing" goals and interventions upon them (i.e., covert rituals undercutting treatment, contributing to the cycling of treatment, lowered belief and efficacy in treatment). It is important to have this conversation in a warm, encouraging, and welcoming manner, underscoring that the door is always open should their position change. Relatedly, CBT-E is not aligned with a goal of weight loss (Fairburn, 2008). We understand that many patients with EDs want to lose weight, but it is important that they know from the start that this treatment is not designed to assist in weight loss or to support the emphasis on weight loss.

Systematic Treatment Protocol

While this book aims to contribute to the literature, it is not a proposed treatment manual. The ideas and suggestions mentioned here are based on extrapolation from the existing literature on OCD and EDs in addition to what we have observed while treating these disorders for many years. However, it is our hope that some of the ideas and points highlighted throughout this text could inspire development of a treatment protocol to be tested empirically.

There are many steps to consider in this process. The first step has been addressed in this book: we have identified the problem and treatment goals and have reviewed the existing literature. We have also consulted with other experts in the field of EDs and OCD. The next step would be to turn the ideas and suggestions mentioned here into a set protocol, or a few versions of a protocol (as goals would differ based on FBT or CBT for the ED portion of treatment). This would involve a step-by-step sequence of procedures to be implemented, in addition to proposed time frames for said procedures. Regarding sequence, the more specificity the better. The next step would be to test the protocol to determine its effectiveness. We expect that perhaps a pilot study or a small case series would come before a randomized controlled trial, as both of those would allow some changes to be made before making the study larger. The very important next step is to evaluate the results to determine if the designed protocol achieved the desired results. The last step would be to use the results to draw implications and then refine the protocol as needed.

In Summary

This chapter aimed to highlight some of the additional considerations for research and practice that apply to this presentation. While the topics mentioned herein are certainly not an exclusive list, they are what we have deemed to be paramount in terms of what the literature is lacking in addition to what clinicians will experience in practice. Regarding the idea of developing a systematic treatment protocol, it is our plan to advocate for this and to be involved in that process in any way we can. In the meantime (and after said protocol is developed) we plan to remain committed to dissemination in the hopes of training as many clinicians as possible in how to best manage co-occurring OCD and EDs.

References

Abramowitz, J. S. (2006). The psychological treatment of obsessive-compulsive disorder. *The Canadian Journal of Psychiatry, 51*(7), 407–416.

Abramowitz, J. S. (2013). The practice of exposure therapy: Relevance of cognitive-behavioral theory and extinction theory. *Behavior Therapy, 44*(4), 548–558.

Abramowitz, J. S., Franklin, M. E., & Cahill, S. P. (2003). Approaches to common obstacles in the exposure-based treatment of obsessive-compulsive disorder. *Cognitive and Behavioral Practice, 10*(1), 14–22.

Abramowitz, J. S., Huppert, J. D., Cohen, A. B., Tolin, D. F., & Cahill, S. P. (2002). Religious obsessions and compulsions in a non-clinical sample: The Penn Inventory of Scrupulosity (PIOS). *Behaviour Research and Therapy, 40*(7), 825–838.

Abramowitz, J. S., & Jacoby, R. J. (2014). Obsessive-compulsive disorder in the DSM-5. *Clinical Psychology: Science and Practice, 21*(3), 221–235.

Abramowitz, J. S., McKay, D., & Taylor, S. (Eds.). (2008). *Clinical handbook of obsessive-compulsive disorder and related problems.* JHU Press.

Accurso, E. C., Lebow, J., Murray, S. B., Kass, A. E., & Le Grange, D. (2016). The relation of weight suppression and BMIz to bulimic symptoms in youth with bulimia nervosa. *Journal of Eating Disorders, 4*(1), 1–6.

Addis, M. E., & Krasnow, A. D. (2000). A national survey of practicing psychologists' attitudes toward psychotherapy treatment manuals. *Journal of Consulting and Clinical Psychology, 68*(2), 331–339.

Agras, W. S., Crow, S. J., Halmi, K. A., et al. (2000). Outcome predictors for the cognitive behavior treatment of bulimia nervosa: Data from a multisite study. *The American Journal of Psychiatry, 157*(8), 1302–1308. https://doi.org/10.1176/appi.ajp.157.8.1302.

Agras, W. S., Rossiter, E. M., Arnow, B., et al. (1992). Pharmacologic and cognitive-behavioral treatment for bulimia nervosa: A controlled comparison. *The American Journal of Psychiatry, 149*(1), 82–87. https://doi.org/10.1176/ajp.149.1.82.

Agras, W. S., Schneider, J. A., Arnow, B., Raeburn, S. D., & Telch, C. F. (1989). Cognitive-behavioral and response-prevention treatments for bulimia nervosa. *Journal of Consulting and Clinical Psychology, 57*(2), 215–221.

Agras, W. S., & Telch, C. F. (1998). The effects of caloric deprivation and negative affect on binge eating in obese binge-eating disordered women. *Behavior Therapy, 29*(3), 491–503.

Agras, W. S., Walsh, T., Fairburn, C. G., Wilson, G. T., & Kraemer, H. C. (2000). A multicenter comparison of cognitive-behavioral therapy and interpersonal psychotherapy for bulimia nervosa. *Archives of General Psychiatry, 57*(5), 459–466. https://doi.org/10.1001/archpsyc.57.5.459.

Albert, U., Venturello, S., Maina, G., Ravizza, L., & Bogetto, F. (2001). Bulimia nervosa with and without obsessive-compulsive syndromes. *Comprehensive Psychiatry, 42*(6), 456–460.

Allan, E., Le Grange, D., Sawyer, S. M., McLean, L. A., & Hughes, E. K. (2018). Parental expressed emotion during two forms of family-based treatment for adolescent anorexia nervosa. *European Eating Disorders Review, 26*(1), 46–52.

Altman, S. E., & Shankman, S. A. (2009). What is the association between obsessive-compulsive disorder and eating disorders? *Clinical Psychology Review, 29*(7), 638–646.

American Psychiatric Association. (2006). Treatment of patients with eating disorders, 3rd ed. American Psychiatric Association. *The American Journal of Psychiatry, 163*(7 Suppl), 4–54.

American Psychiatric Association. (2013). *Diagnostic and statistical manual of mental disorders* (5th ed.). American Psychiatric Association.

Anestis, M. D., Selby, E. A., Fink, E. L., & Joiner, T. E. (2007). The multifaceted role of distress tolerance in dysregulated eating behaviors. *International Journal of Eating Disorders, 40*(8), 718–726.

Angst, J., Gamma, A., Endrass, J. et al. (2004). Obsessive-compulsive severity spectrum in the community: Prevalence, comorbidity, and course. *European Archives of Psychiatry and Clinical Neurosciences 254*, 156–164. https://doi.org/10.1007/s00406-0 04-0459-4.

Ashby, J. S., & Bruner, L. P. (2005). Multidimensional perfectionism and obsessive-compulsive behaviors. *Journal of College Counseling, 8*(1), 31–40.

Atiye, M., Miettunen, J., & Raevuori-Helkamaa, A. (2015). A meta-analysis of temperament in eating disorders. *European Eating Disorders Review, 23*(2), 89–99. https://doi.org/10.1002 /erv.2342.

Balci, V., & Sevincok, L. (2010). Suicidal ideation in patients with obsessive-compulsive disorder. *Psychiatry Research, 175*(1–2), 104–108. https://doi.org/10.1016/j .psychres.2009.03.012.

Bang, L., Kristensen, U. B., Wisting, L. et al. (2020). Presence of eating disorder symptoms in patients with obsessive-compulsive disorder. *BMC Psychiatry 20*, 36. https://doi.org/10.1186/s1 2888-020-2457-0.

Baracos, V. E. (2001). A deadly combination of anorexia and hypermetabolism. *Current Opinion in Clinical Nutrition & Metabolic Care, 4*(3), 175–177.

Bardone-Cone, A. M., Wonderlich, S. A., Frost, R. O., et al. (2007). Perfectionism and eating disorders: Current status and future directions. *Clinical Psychology Review, 27*(3), 384–405.

Barreto, M., & Ellemers, N. (2005). The burden of benevolent sexism: How it contributes to the maintenance of gender inequalities. *European Journal of Social Psychology, 35*(3), 633–642.

Barrett, P., Healy-Farrell, L., & March, J. S. (2004). Cognitive-behavioral family treatment of childhood obsessive-compulsive disorder: A controlled trial. *Journal of the American Academy of Child and Adolescent Psychiatry, 43*(1), 46–62. https://doi.org/10 .1097/00004583-200401000-00014.

Beadle, J. N., Paradiso, S., Salerno, A., & McCormick, L. M. (2013). Alexithymia, emotional empathy, and self-regulation in anorexia nervosa. *Annals of Clinical Psychiatry: Official Journal of the American Academy of Clinical Psychiatrists, 25*(2), 107–120.

Beck, A. T. (1979). *Cognitive therapy and the emotional disorders.* Penguin.

Becker, C. B., Farrell, N. R., & Waller, G. (2020). *Exposure therapy for eating disorders.* Oxford University Press.

Becker, C. B., & Waller, G. (2017). The use of exposure-based strategies in treating eating disorders. In T. Wade (Eds.), *Encyclopedia of Feeding and Eating Disorders* (pp. 378–383). Springer.

Becker, C. B., Zayfert, C., & Anderson, E. (2004a). A survey of psychologists' attitudes towards and utilization of exposure therapy for PTSD. *Behaviour Research and Therapy, 42*(3), 277–292.

Becker, D. J., Zayfert, C., & Anderson, E. (2004b). Clinician attitudes toward exposure therapy: A survey of anxiety disorder specialists. *Behaviour Research and Therapy, 42*(9), 1115–1122.

Bello, N. T., & Hajnal, A. (2010). Dopamine and binge eating behaviors. *Pharmacology Biochemistry and Behavior, 97*(1), 25–33.

Belloch, A., Roncero, M., & Perpiñá, C. (2016). Obsessional and eating disorder-related intrusive thoughts: Differences and similarities within and between individuals vulnerable to OCD or to EDs. *European Eating Disorders Review, 24*(6), 446–454.

Bellodi, L., Cavallini, M. C., Bertelli, S., et al. (2001). Morbidity risk for obsessive-compulsive spectrum disorders in first-degree relatives of patients with eating disorders. *American Journal of Psychiatry, 158*(4), 563–569.

Benito, K. G., & Walther, M. (2015). Therapeutic process during exposure: Habituation model. *Journal of Obsessive-Compulsive and Related Disorders*, 6, 147–157.

Berle, D., & Starcevic, V. (2005). Thought–action fusion: Review of the literature and future directions. *Clinical Psychology Review*, 25(3), 263–284.

Berman, N. C., Wheaton, M. G., McGrath, P., & Abramowitz, J. S. (2010). Predicting anxiety: The role of experiential avoidance and anxiety sensitivity. *Journal of Anxiety Disorders*, 24(1), 109–113.

Berner, L. A., Shaw, J. A., Witt, A. A., & Lowe, M. R. (2013). The relation of weight suppression and body mass index to symptomatology and treatment response in anorexia nervosa. *Journal of Abnormal Psychology*, 122(3), 694.

Bernstein, A., Zvolensky, M. J., Vujanovic, A. A., & Moos, R. (2009). Integrating anxiety sensitivity, distress tolerance, and discomfort intolerance: A hierarchical model of affect sensitivity and tolerance. *Behavior Therapy*, 40(3), 291–301.

Besiroglu, L., Uguz, F., Saglam, M., Agargun, M. Y., & Cilli, A. S. (2007). Factors associated with major depressive disorder occurring after the onset of obsessive-compulsive disorder. *Journal of Affective Disorders*, 102(1–3), 73–79.

Birrell, J., Meares, K., Wilkinson, A., & Freeston, M. (2011). Toward a definition of intolerance of uncertainty: A review of factor analytical studies of the Intolerance of Uncertainty Scale. *Clinical Psychology Review*, 31(7), 1198–1208.

Bodell, L. P., & Keel, P. K. (2015). Weight suppression in bulimia nervosa: Associations with biology and behavior. *Journal of Abnormal Psychology*, 124(4), 994.

Bodell, L. P., Racine, S. E., & Wildes, J. E. (2016). Examining weight suppression as a predictor of eating disorder symptom trajectories in anorexia nervosa. *International Journal of Eating Disorders*, 49(8), 753–763.

Boger, S., Ehring, T., Berberich, G., & Werner, G. G. (2020). Impact of childhood maltreatment on obsessive-compulsive disorder symptom severity and treatment outcome. *European Journal of Psychotraumatology*, 11(1), 1753942.

Bottesi, G., Ghisi, M., Sica, C., & Freeston, M. H. (2017). Intolerance of uncertainty, not just right experiences, and compulsive checking: Test of a moderated mediation model on a non-clinical sample. *Comprehensive Psychiatry*, 73, 111–119.

Boudewyns, P. A., & Shipley, R. H. (1983). Direct therapeutic exposure. In *Flooding and implosive therapy* (pp. 1–14). Springer.

Bouton, M. E. (1993). Context, time, and memory retrieval in the interference paradigms of Pavlovian learning. *Psychological Bulletin*, 114(1), 80.

Bragdon, L. B., & Coles, M. E. (2017). Examining heterogeneity of obsessive-compulsive disorder: Evidence for subgroups based on motivations. *Journal of Anxiety Disorders*, 45, 64–71.

Bratman, S. (1997). Orthorexia nervosa. *Yoga Journal*, 136, 42–50.

Brockmeyer, T., Holtforth, M. G., Bents, H., et al. (2012). Starvation and emotion regulation in anorexia nervosa. *Comprehensive Psychiatry*, 53(5), 496–501.

Brody, E. M., & Kleban, M. H. (1981). Physical and mental health symptoms of older people: Who do they tell? *Journal of the American Geriatrics Society*, 29(10), 442–449.

Brown, R. A., & Lewinsohn, P. M. (1984). A psychoeducational approach to the treatment of depression: Comparison of group, individual, and minimal contact procedures. *Journal of Consulting and Clinical Psychology*, 52(5), 774.

Brownley, K. A., Berkman, N. D., Sedway, J. A., et al. (2007). Binge eating disorder treatment: A systematic review of randomized controlled trials. *The International Journal of Eating Disorders*, 40(4), 337–348. https://doi.org/10.1002/eat.20370.

Buckner, J. D., Keough, M. E., & Schmidt, N. B. (2007). Problematic alcohol and cannabis use among young adults: The roles of depression and discomfort and distress tolerance. *Addictive Behaviors*, 32(9), 1957–1963.

Bulik, C. M., Carroll, I. M., & Mehler, P. (2021). Reframing anorexia nervosa as a metabo-psychiatric disorder. *Trends in Endocrinology & Metabolism, 32*(10), 752–761.

Bulik, C. M., Sullivan, P. F., Carter, F. A., et al. (1998). The role of exposure with response prevention in the cognitive-behavioural therapy for bulimia nervosa. *Psychological Medicine, 28*(3), 611–623.

Butryn, M. L., Lowe, M. R., Safer, D. L., & Agras, W. S. (2006). Weight suppression is a robust predictor of outcome in the cognitive-behavioral treatment of bulimia nervosa. *Journal of Abnormal Psychology, 115* (1), 62.

Byrne, S., Wade, T., Hay, P., et al. (2017). A randomised controlled trial of three psychological treatments for anorexia nervosa. *Psychological Medicine, 47*(16), 2823–2833. https://doi.org/10.1017 /S0033291717001349.

Calamari, J. E., & Cassiday, K. L. (1999). Treating obsessive-compulsive disorder in older adults: A review of strategies. In M. Duffy (Ed.), Handbook of counseling and psychotherapy with older adults (pp. 526 -538). John Wiley & Sons, Inc.

Carmin, C. N., & Wiegartz, P. S. (2000). Successful and unsuccessful treatment of obsessive-compulsive disorder in older adults. *Journal of Contemporary Psychotherapy, 30*(2), 181–193.

Carter, F. A., McIntosh, V. V., Joyce, P. R., Sullivan, P. F., & Bulik, C. M. (2003). Role of exposure with response prevention in cognitive-behavioral therapy for bulimia nervosa: Three-year follow-up results. *International Journal of Eating Disorders, 33* (2), 127–135.

Carter, R. T., Johnson, V. E., Kirkinis, K., et al. (2019). A meta-analytic review of racial discrimination: Relationships to health and culture. *Race and Social Problems, 11*(1), 15–32.

Casper R. C. (1990). Personality features of women with good outcome from restricting anorexia nervosa. *Psychosomatic Medicine, 52* (2), 156–170. https://doi.org/10.1097/000068 42-199003000-00004.

Cassioli, E., Sensi, C., Mannucci, E., Ricca, V., & Rotella, F. (2020). Pharmacological treatment of acute-phase anorexia nervosa: Evidence from randomized controlled trials. *Journal of Psychopharmacology, 34*(8), 864–873. https:// doi.org/10.1177/0269881120920453.

Cassin, S. E., & von Ranson, K. M. (2005). Personality and eating disorders: A decade in review. *Clinical Psychology Review, 25*(7), 895–916.

Catapano, F., Perris, F., Fabrazzo, M., et al. (2010). Obsessive-compulsive disorder with poor insight: A three-year prospective study. *Progress in Neuro-Psychopharmacology and Biological Psychiatry, 34*(2), 323–330.

Çelikel, F.C., Bingol, T.Y., Yıldırım, D., Tel, H., & Erkorkmaz, U. (2009). Eating attitudes in patients with obsessive compulsive disorder. *Archives of Neuropsychiatry, 46*, 86–90.

Chambless, D. L., Baker, M.J., Baucom, D. H., et al. (1998). Update on empirically validated therapies, II. *The Clinical Psychologist, 51*, 3–16.

Champion, L. & Power, M. (2012). Interpersonal psychotherapy for eating disorders. *Clinical Psychology and Psychotherapy, 19*(2), 150–158. https://doi.org/10.1002/cpp.1780.

Channon, S., De Silva, P., Hemsley, D., & Perkins, R. (1989). A controlled trial of cognitive-behavioural and behavioural treatment of anorexia nervosa. *Behaviour Research and Therapy, 27*(5), 529–535.

Chen, E. Y., Matthews, L., Allen, C., Kuo, J. R., & Linehan, M. M. (2008). Dialectical behavior therapy for clients with binge-eating disorder or bulimia nervosa and borderline personality disorder. *The International Journal of Eating Disorders, 41*(6), 505–512. https://doi.org/10.1002/eat.20522.

Christie, D., Watkins, B., & Lask, B. (2000). Assessment. In R. Bryant-Waugh & B. Lask, *Anorexia nervosa and related eating disorders in childhood and adolescence* (2nd ed., pp. 105–126). Psychology Press.

Clark, D. A. (2005). Focus on "cognition" in cognitive behavior therapy for OCD: Is it really necessary? *Cognitive Behaviour Therapy, 34*(3), 131–139.

Clark, D. A. (2020). *Cognitive-behavioral therapy for OCD and its subtypes.* Guilford Publications.

Cochrane, C. E., Brewerton, T. D., Wilson, D. B., & Hodges, E. L. (1993). Alexithymia in the eating disorders. *International Journal of Eating Disorders, 14*(2), 219–222.

Coffino, J. A., Udo, T., & Grilo, C. M. (2019a). The significance of overvaluation of shape or weight in binge-eating disorder: Results from a national sample of US adults. *Obesity (Silver Spring, Md.)*, 27(8), 1367–1371. https://doi.org/10.1002/oby.22539.

Coffino, J. A., Udo, T., & Grilo, C. M. (2019b). Rates of help-seeking in US adults with lifetime DSM-5 eating disorders: Prevalence across diagnoses and differences by sex and ethnicity/race. *Mayo Clinic Proceedings*, 94(8), 1415–1426. https://doi.org/10.1016/j.mayocp.2019.02.030.

Conway, C. C., Naragon-Gainey, K., & Harris, M. T. (2021). The structure of distress tolerance and neighboring emotion regulation abilities. *Assessment*, 28(4), 1050–1064.

Cooper, M., Cohen-Tovée, E., Todd, G., Wells, A., & Tovée, M. (1997). The eating disorder belief questionnaire: Preliminary development. *Behaviour Research and Therapy*, 35(4), 381–388. https://doi.org/10.1016/s0005-7967(96)00115-5.

Cooper, Z., & Fairburn, C. (1987). The eating disorder examination: A semi-structured interview for the assessment of the specific psychopathology of eating disorders. *International Journal of Eating Disorders*, 6(1), 1–8.

Cooper, Z., & Fairburn, C. G. (2011). The evolution of "enhanced" cognitive behavior therapy for eating disorders: Learning from treatment nonresponse. *Cognitive and Behavioral Practice*, 18(3), 394–402. https://doi.org/10.1016/j.cbpra.2010.07.007.

Cooper, M., & Kelland, H. (2015). Medication and psychotherapy in eating disorders: Is there a gap between research and practice? *Journal of Eating Disorders*, 3, 45. https://doi.org/10.1186/s40337-015-0080-0.

Cooper, Z., & Stewart, I. (2008). CBT-E and the younger patient. In C. G. Fairburn, Z. Cooper, R. Shafran, & G. T. Wilson (Eds.), *Eating disorders: A transdiagnostic protocol* (pp. 221–234). Routledge

Cottraux, J., Note, I., Yao, S. N., et al. (2001). A randomized controlled trial of cognitive therapy versus intensive behavior therapy in obsessive compulsive disorder. *Psychotherapy and Psychosomatics*, 70(6), 288–297.

Corstorphine, E. (2006). Cognitive–emotional–behavioural therapy for the eating disorders: Working with beliefs about emotions. *European Eating Disorders Review: The Professional Journal of the Eating Disorders Association*, 14(6), 448–461.

Corstorphine, E., Mountford, V., Tomlinson, S., Waller, G., & Meyer, C. (2007). Distress tolerance in the eating disorders. *Eating Behaviors*, 8(1), 91–97.

Cougle, J. R., Timpano, K. R., Fitch, K. E., & Hawkins, K. A. (2011). Distress tolerance and obsessions: An integrative analysis. *Depression and Anxiety*, 28(10), 906–914.

Cougle, J. R., Timpano, K. R., & Goetz, A. R. (2012). Exploring the unique and interactive roles of distress tolerance and negative urgency in obsessions. *Personality and Individual Differences*, 52(4), 515–520.

Cougle, J. R., Timpano, K. R., Sarawgi, S., Smith, C. M., & Fitch, K. E. (2013). A multi-modal investigation of the roles of distress tolerance and emotional reactivity in obsessive-compulsive symptoms. *Anxiety, Stress & Coping*, 26(5), 478–492.

Cournoyer, L. G., Brochu, S., Landry, M., & Bergeron, J. (2007). Therapeutic alliance, patient behaviour and dropout in a drug rehabilitation programme: The moderating effect of clinical subpopulations. *Addiction*, 102(12), 1960–1970.

Craske, M. (2015). Optimizing exposure therapy for anxiety disorders: An inhibitory learning and inhibitory regulation approach. *Verhaltenstherapie*, 25(2), 134–143.

Craske, M. G., Kircanski, K., Zelikowsky, M., et al. (2008). Optimizing inhibitory learning during exposure therapy. *Behaviour Research and Therapy*, 46(1), 5–27.

Craske, M. G., Treanor, M., Conway, C. C., Zbozinek, T., & Vervliet, B. (2014). Maximizing exposure therapy: An inhibitory learning approach. *Behaviour Research and Therapy*, 58, 10–23. http://dx.doi.org/10.1016/j.brat.2014.04.006.

Crino, R. D., & Andrews, G. (1996). Obsessive-compulsive disorder and axis I comorbidity. *Journal of Anxiety Disorders*, 10(1), 37–46.

Crow, S. J., Swanson, S. A., Le Grange, D., Feig, E. H., & Merikangas, K. R. (2014). Suicidal behavior in adolescents and adults with bulimia nervosa. *Comprehensive Psychiatry*, 55(7), 1534–1539

Curtis, V., De Barra, M., & Aunger, R. (2011). Disgust as an adaptive system for disease avoidance behaviour. *Philosophical Transactions of the Royal Society B: Biological Sciences*, 366(1563), 389–401.

da Conceição Costa, D. L., Shavitt, R. G., Cesar, R. C. C., et al. (2013). Can early improvement be an indicator of treatment response in obsessive-compulsive disorder? Implications for early-treatment decision-making. *Journal of Psychiatric Research*, 47(11), 1700–1707.

Dalle Grave, A., & Sapuppo, W. (2020). Treatment of avoidant/restrictive food intake disorder: A systematic review. *Italian Journal of Eating Disorders and Obesity*, 4, 13–23.

Dalle Grave, R., Calugi, S., Doll, H. A., & Fairburn, C. G. (2013). Enhanced cognitive behaviour therapy for adolescents with anorexia nervosa: An alternative to family therapy? *Behaviour Research and Therapy*, 51(1), R9–R12. https://doi.org/10.1016/j.brat.2012.09.008.

Dalle Grave, R., Calugi, S., & Marchesini, G. (2008). Is amenorrhea a clinically useful criterion for the diagnosis of anorexia nervosa? *Behaviour Research and Therapy*, 46(12), 1290–1294.

Dalle Grave, R., Eckhardt, S., Calugi, S., & Le Grange, D. (2019). A conceptual comparison of family-based treatment and enhanced cognitive behavior therapy in the treatment of adolescents with eating disorders. *Journal of Eating Disorders*, 7, 42. https://doi.org/10.1186/s40337-019-0275-x.

Dalle Grave, R., El Ghoch, M., Sartirana, M., & Calugi, S. (2016). Cognitive behavioral therapy for anorexia nervosa: An update. *Current Psychiatry Reports*, 18(1), 2. https://doi.org/10.1007/s11920-015-0643-4.

Daughters, S. B., Lejuez, C. W., Strong, D. R., et al. (2005). The relationship among negative affect, distress tolerance, and length of gambling abstinence attempt. *Journal of Gambling Studies*, 21, 363–378.

Daughters, S. B., Sargeant, M. N., Bornovalova, M. A., Gratz, K. L., & Lejuez, C. W. (2008). The relationship between distress tolerance and antisocial personality disorder among male inner-city treatment seeking substance users. *Journal of Personality Disorders*, 22(5), 509–524.

Deacon, B. J., & Abramowitz, J. (2006). Anxiety sensitivity and its dimensions across the anxiety disorders. *Journal of Anxiety Disorders*, 20(7), 837–857.

Deacon, B. J., & Farrell, N. R. (2013). Therapist barriers to the dissemination of exposure therapy. In D. McKay, & E. Storch (Eds.), *Handbook of treating variants and complications in anxiety disorders*. Springer Press.

Deacon, B. J., Farrell, N. R., Kemp, J. J., et al. (2013). Assessing therapist reservations about exposure therapy for anxiety disorders: The Therapist Beliefs about Exposure Scale. *Journal of Anxiety Disorders*, 27(8), 772–780.

DeMarco, R. M., & Sell, R. L. (2015). Exploring the relationship between LGBTQ+ identity and disordered eating. *Journal of Homosexuality*, 62(6), 835–854.

Denys, D., Tenney, N., van Megen, H. J., de Geus, F., & Westenberg, H. G. (2004). Axis I and II comorbidity in a large sample of patients with obsessive-compulsive disorder. *Journal of Affective Disorders*, 80(2–3), 155–162.

DiBartolo, P. M., Li, C. Y., & Frost, R. O. (2008). How do the dimensions of perfectionism relate to mental health? *Cognitive Therapy and Research*, 32(3), 401–417.

Diefenbach, G. J., Abramowitz, J. S., Norberg, M. M., & Tolin, D. F. (2007). Changes in quality of life following cognitive-behavioral therapy for obsessive-compulsive disorder. *Behaviour Research and Therapy*, 45(12), 3060–3068.

Dixon, J. B., Egger, G. J., Finkelstein, E. A., Kral, J. G., & Lambert, G. W. (2015). "Obesity paradox" misunderstands the biology of optimal weight throughout the life cycle. *International Journal of Obesity*, 39(1), 82–84.

Donker, T., Griffiths, K. M., Cuijpers, P., & Christensen, H. (2009). Psychoeducation for depression, anxiety and psychological distress: A meta-analysis. *BMC Medicine*, 7(1), 1–9.

Doron, G., Kyrios, M., & Moulding, R. (2007). Sensitive domains of self-concept in obsessive-compulsive disorder (OCD): Further evidence for a multidimensional model of OCD. *Journal of Anxiety Disorders, 21*(3), 433–444.

Doron, G., Sar-El, D., & Mikulincer, M. (2012). Threats to moral self-perceptions trigger obsessive compulsive contamination-related behavioral tendencies. *Journal of Behavior Therapy and Experimental Psychiatry, 43*(3), 884–890.

Doyle, P., Le Grange, D., Celio-Doyle, A., Loeb, K., & Crosby, R. (2010). Early response to family-based treatment for adolescent anorexia nervosa. *International Journal of Eating Disorders, 43,* 659–662

D'Souza, R., McEvoy, P. M., & Rapee, R. M. (2019). Therapists' attitudes toward and use of exposure therapy: A systematic review. *Clinical Psychology Review, 66,* 1–16.

D'Souza Walsh, K., Davies, L., Pluckwell, H., Huffinley, H., & Waller, G. (2019). Alliance, technique, both, or more? Clinicians' views on what works in cognitive-behavioral therapy for eating disorders. *International Journal of Eating Disorders, 52*(3), 278–282.

Dugas, M. J., Gagnon, F., Ladouceur, R., & Freeston, M. H. (1998). Generalized anxiety disorder: A preliminary test of a conceptual model. *Behaviour Research and Therapy, 36* (2), 215–226.

Dugas, M. J., Gosselin, P., & Ladouceur, R. (2001). Intolerance of uncertainty and worry: Investigating specificity in a nonclinical sample. *Cognitive Therapy and Research, 25,* 551–558.

Dunn, T. M., & Bratman, S. (2016). On orthorexia nervosa: A review of the literature and proposed diagnostic criteria. *Eating Behaviors, 21,* 11–17.

Durso, L. E., Latner, J. D., White, M. A., et al. (2012). Internalized weight bias in obese patients with binge ED: Associations with eating disturbances and psychological functioning. *International Journal of Eating Disorders, 45*(3), 423–427.

Eddy, K. T., Dutra, L., Bradley, R., & Westen, D. (2004). A multidimensional meta-analysis of psychotherapy and pharmacotherapy for obsessive-compulsive disorder. *Clinical Psychology Review, 24*(8), 1011–1030.

Edelmann, R. J. (1987). *The psychology of embarrassment.* John Wiley & Sons.

Ehrlich, S., Burghardt, R., Weiss, D., et al. (2008). Glial and neuronal damage markers in patients with anorexia nervosa. *Journal of Neural Transmission, 115*(6), 921–927.

Eifert, G. H., & Heffner, M. (2003). The effects of acceptance versus control contexts on avoidance of panic-related symptoms. *Journal of Behavior Therapy and Experimental Psychiatry, 34*(3–4), 293–312.

Elsesser, K. M. (2016). Gender bias against female leaders: A review. In M. Connerley & J. Wu (Eds.), *Handbook on well-being of working women* (pp. 161–173). Springer.

Elsner, B., Jacobi, T., Kischkel, E., Schulze, D., & Reuter, B. (2022). Mechanisms of exposure and response prevention in obsessive-compulsive disorder: Effects of habituation and expectancy violation on short-term outcome in cognitive behavioral therapy. *BMC Psychiatry, 22*(1), 1–16.

Erol, A., Toprak, G., & Yazici, F. (2002). Predicting factors of eating disorders and general psychological symptoms in female college students. *Turk psikiyatri dergisi [Turkish Journal of Psychiatry], 13*(1), 48–57.

Erskine, H. E., & Whiteford, H. A. (2018). Epidemiology of binge eating disorder. *Current Opinion in Psychiatry, 31*(6), 462–470.

Fairburn, C. G. (2008). *Cognitive behavior therapy and eating disorders.* Guilford Press.

Fairburn, C. G. (2013). *Overcoming binge eating: The proven program to learn why you binge and how you can stop.* Guilford press.

Fairburn, C. G., Agras, W. S., Walsh, B. T., Wilson, G. T., & Stice, E. (2004). Prediction of outcome in bulimia nervosa by early change in treatment. *The American Journal of Psychiatry, 161*(12), 2322–2324. https://doi.org/10.1176/appi.ajp.161.12.2322.

Fairburn, C. G., Bailey-Straebler, S., Basden, S., et al. (2015). A transdiagnostic comparison of enhanced cognitive behaviour therapy (CBT-E) and interpersonal psychotherapy in the treatment of eating disorders. *Behaviour*

Research and Therapy, 70, 64–71. https://doi .org/10.1016/j.brat.2015.04.010.

Fairburn, C. G., Cooper, Z., Doll, H. A., et al. (2009). Transdiagnostic cognitive-behavioral therapy for patients with eating disorders: A two-site trial with 60-week follow-up. *American Journal of Psychiatry, 166*(3), 311–319.

Fairburn, C. G., Cooper, Z., Doll, H. A., et al. (2013). Enhanced cognitive behaviour therapy for adults with anorexia nervosa: A UK–Italy study. *Behaviour Research and Therapy, 51*(1), R2–R8. https://doi.org/10 .1016/j.brat.2012.09.010.

Fairburn, C. G., Cooper, Z., Shafran, R. (2003). Cognitive behaviour therapy for eating disorders: A "transdiagnostic" theory and treatment. *Behaviour Research and Therapy,* 41, 509–528.

Fairburn, C. G., Jones, R., Peveler, R. C., Hope, R. A., & O'Connor, M. (1993). Psychotherapy and bulimia nervosa: Longer-term effects of interpersonal psychotherapy, behavior therapy, and cognitive behavior therapy. *Archives of General Psychiatry, 50*(6), 419–428.

Fals-Stewart, W., Marks, A. P., & Schafer, J. (1993). A comparison of behavioral group therapy and individual behavior therapy in treating obsessive-compulsive disorder. *Journal of Nervous and Mental Disease, 181* (3), 189–193.

Farrell, N. R., Bowie, O. R., Cimperman, M. M., et al. (2019). Exploring the preliminary effectiveness and acceptability of food-based exposure therapy for eating disorders: A case series of adult inpatients. *Journal of Experimental Psychopathology, 10*(1), 2043808718824886.

Farrell, N. R., Deacon, B. J., Dixon, L. J., & Lickel, J. J. (2013). Theory-based training strategies for modifying practitioner concerns about exposure therapy. *Journal of Anxiety Disorders, 27*(8), 781–787.

Fineberg, N. A., Reghunandanan, S., Brown, A., & Pampaloni, I. (2013). Pharmacotherapy of obsessive-compulsive disorder: Evidence-based treatment and beyond. *The Australian and New Zealand Journal of Psychiatry, 47*(2), 121–141. https://doi.org/10 .1177/0004867412461958.

First, M. B., Williams, J. B. W., Karg, R. S., & Spitzer, R. L. (2016). *User's guide for the SCID-5-CV Structured Clinical Interview for DSM-5® disorders: Clinical version.* American Psychiatric Publishing, Inc.

Fisher, P. L., & Wells, A. (2005). How effective are cognitive and behavioral treatments for obsessive-compulsive disorder? A clinical significance analysis. *Behaviour Research and Therapy, 43*(12), 1543–1558.

Flament, M. F., Bissada, H., & Spettigue, W. (2012). Evidence-based pharmacotherapy of eating disorders. *The International Journal of Neuropsychopharmacology, 15*(2), 189–207. https://doi.org/10.1017/S1461145711000381.

Flegal, K. M., Kit, B. K., Orpana, H., & Graubard, B. I. (2013). Association of all-cause mortality with overweight and obesity using standard body mass index categories: A systematic review and meta-analysis. *JAMA, 309*(1), 71–82.

Flygare, O., Andersson, E., Ringberg, H., et al. (2020). Adapted cognitive behavior therapy for obsessive-compulsive disorder with co-occurring autism spectrum disorder: A clinical effectiveness study. *Autism, 24*(1), 190–199.

Foa, E. B. (2010). Cognitive behavioral therapy of obsessive-compulsive disorder. *Dialogues in Clinical Neuroscience, 12,* 199–207.

Foa, E. B., Abramowitz, J. S., Franklin, M. E., & Kozak, M. J. (1999). Feared consequences, fixity of belief, and treatment outcome in patients with obsessive-compulsive disorder. *Behavior Therapy, 30*(4), 717–724.

Foa, E. B., & Kozak, M. J. (1986). Emotional processing of fear: Exposure to corrective information. *Psychological Bulletin, 99* (1), 20.

Foa, E. B., Liebowitz, M. R., Kozak, M. J., et al. (2005). Randomized, placebo-controlled trial of exposure and ritual prevention, clomipramine, and their combination in the treatment of obsessive-compulsive disorder. *American Journal of Psychiatry, 162*(1), 151–161.

Foa, E. B., Steketee, G., Grayson, J. B., & Docherty, J. P. (1997). *A cognitive-behavioral treatment manual: Obsessive-compulsive disorder.*

Fontana, A., Rosenheck, R., & Spencer, R. A. (1993). *The long journey home, III: Third progress report on the specialized PTSD programs. Northeast Program Evaluation Center.*

Fornés-Romero, G., & Belloch, A. (2017). Induced not just right and incompleteness experiences in OCD patients and non-clinical individuals: An in vivo study. *Journal of Behavior Therapy and Experimental Psychiatry, 57,* 103–112.

Fourtounas, A., & Thomas, S. J. (2016). Cognitive factors predicting checking, procrastination and other maladaptive behaviours: Prospective versus inhibitory intolerance of uncertainty. *Journal of Obsessive-Compulsive and Related Disorders, 9,* 30–35.

Frank, G. K. (2014). Could dopamine agonists aid in drug development for anorexia nervosa? *Frontiers in Nutrition, 1,* 19.

Frank, G. K., & Kaye, W. H. (2012). Current status of functional imaging in eating disorders. *International Journal of Eating Disorders, 45*(6), 723–736.

Freeman, C. P. L., Barry, F., Dunkeld-Turnbull, J., & Henderson, A. (1988). Controlled trial of psychotherapy for bulimia nervosa. *British Medical Journal (Clinical Research Edition), 296*(6621), 521–525.

Freeston, M. H., Ladouceur, R., Gagnon, F., et al. (1997). Cognitive-behavioral treatment of obsessive thoughts: A controlled study. *Journal of Consulting and Clinical Psychology, 65*(3), 405.

Fullana, M. A., Vilagut, G., Rojas-Farreras, S., et al. (2010). Obsessive-compulsive symptom dimensions in the general population: Results from an epidemiological study in six European countries. *Journal of Affective Disorders, 124*(3), 291–299.

Galmiche, M., Déchelotte, P., Lambert, G., & Tavolacci, M.P. (2019). Prevalence of eating disorders over the 2000–2018 period: A systematic literature review. *The American Journal of Clinical Nutrition, 109*(5), 1402–1413. https://doi.org/10.1093/ajcn/nqy342.

Garber, A. K., Mauldin, K., Michihata, N., et al. (2013). Higher calorie diets increase rate of weight gain and shorten hospital stay in hospitalized adolescents with anorexia nervosa. *Journal of Adolescent Health, 53*(5), 579–584.

García-Soriano, G., & Belloch, A. (2012). Exploring the role of obsessive-compulsive relevant self-worth contingencies in obsessive-compulsive disorder patients. *Psychiatry Research, 198*(1), 94–99.

Garcia, A. M., Sapyta, J. J., Moore, P. S., et al. (2010). Predictors and moderators of treatment outcome in the Pediatric Obsessive Compulsive Treatment Study (POTS I). *Journal of the American Academy of Child & Adolescent Psychiatry, 49*(10), 1024–1033.

García-Soriano, G., Roncero, M., Perpiñá, C., & Belloch, A. (2014). Intrusive thoughts in obsessive-compulsive disorder and eating disorder patients: A differential analysis. *European Eating Disorders Review, 22*(3), 191–199.

Gardenghi, G. G., Boni, E., Todisco, P., et al. (2009). Respiratory function in patients with stable anorexia nervosa. *Chest, 136*(5), 1356–1363.

Garner, D. M., & Garfinkel, P. E. (Eds.). (1997). *Handbook of treatment for eating disorders.* Guilford Press.

Gay, P., Schmidt, R. E., & Van der Linden, M. (2011). Impulsivity and intrusive thoughts: Related manifestations of self-control difficulties? *Cognitive Therapy and Research, 35,* 293–303.

Geller, J., Cassin, S. E., Brown, K. E., & Srikameswaran, S. (2009). Factors associated with improvements in readiness for change: Low vs. normal BMI eating disorders. *International Journal of Eating Disorders, 42*(1), 40–46.

Geller, J., & Dunn, E. C. (2011). Integrating motivational interviewing and cognitive behavioral therapy in the treatment of eating disorders: Tailoring interventions to patient readiness for change. *Cognitive and Behavioral Practice, 18*(1), 5–15.

Geller, J., & Srikameswaran, S. (2015). What effective therapies have in common. *Advances in Eating Disorders: Theory, Research and Practice, 3*(2), 191–197.

Gentes, E. L., & Ruscio, A. M. (2011). A meta-analysis of the relation of intolerance of uncertainty to symptoms of generalized anxiety disorder, major depressive disorder, and obsessive-compulsive disorder. *Clinical Psychology Review, 31*(6), 923–933.

George, L., Thornton, C., Touyz, S. W., Waller, G., & Beumont, P. J. (2004). Motivational enhancement and schema-focused cognitive behaviour therapy in the treatment of chronic eating disorders. *Clinical Psychologist, 8*(2), 81–85.

Gianini, L., Liu, Y., Wang, Y., et al. (2015). Abnormal eating behavior in video-recorded meals in anorexia nervosa. *Eating Behaviors, 19*, 28–32. https://doi.org/10.1016/j.eatbeh.2015.06.005.

Gillihan, S. J., Williams, M. T., Malcoun, E., Yadin, E., & Foa, E. B. (2012). Common pitfalls in exposure and response prevention (EX/RP) for OCD. *Journal of Obsessive-Compulsive and Related Disorders, 1*(4), 251–257.

Godart, N. T., Flament, M. F., Perdereau, F., & Jeammet, P. (2002). Comorbidity between eating disorders and anxiety disorders: A review. *International Journal of Eating Disorders, 32*(3), 253–270.

Godart, N. T., Flament, M. F., Curt, F., et al. (2003). Anxiety disorders in subjects seeking treatment for eating disorders: A DSM-IV controlled study. *Psychiatry Research, 117*(3), 245–258.

Godier, L. R., & Park, R. J. (2014). Compulsivity in anorexia nervosa: A transdiagnostic concept. *Frontiers in Psychology, 5*, 778.

Goldner, E. M., Cockell, S. J., & Srikameswaran, S. (2002). Perfectionism and eating disorders. In G. L. Flett & P. L. Hewitt (Eds.), *Perfectionism: Theory, research, and treatment* (pp. 319–340). American Psychological Association. https://doi.org/10.1037/10458-013.

Goldstein, D. J., Wilson, M. G., Thompson, V. L., Potvin, J. H., & Rampey, A. H., Jr. (1995). Long-term fluoxetine treatment of bulimia nervosa. Fluoxetine Bulimia Nervosa Research Group. *The British Journal of Psychiatry: The Journal of Mental Science, 166*(5), 660–666. https://doi.org/10.1192/bjp.166.5.660.

Goodman, W. K., Price, L. H., Rasmussen, S. A., et al. (1989). The Yale–Brown obsessive compulsive scale: I. Development, use, and reliability. *Archives of General Psychiatry, 46*(11), 1006–1011.

Gordon, A. R., Moore, L. B., & Guss, C. (2021). Eating disorders among transgender and gender non-binary people. In *Eating disorders in boys and men* (pp. 265–281). Springer.

Graber, J. A., & Brooks-Gunn, J. (2001). Co-occurring eating and depressive problems: An 8-year study of adolescent girls. *International Journal of Eating Disorders, 30*(1), 37–47.

Gratz, K. L., Rosenthal, M. Z., Tull, M. T., Lejuez, C. W., & Gunderson, J. G. (2006). An experimental investigation of emotion dysregulation in borderline personality disorder. *Journal of Abnormal Psychology, 115*(4), 850.

Grayson, J. B., Foa, E. B., & Steketee, G. (1982). Habituation during exposure treatment: Distraction vs attention-focusing. *Behaviour Research and Therapy, 20*(4), 323–328.

Greenberg, D., Witzum, E., Pato, M. T., & Zohar, J. (2001). Treatment of strictly religious patients. In M. T. Pato & J. Zohar (Eds.), *Current treatments of obsessive-compulsive disorder* (pp. 173–191). American Psychiatric Association.

Grilo, C. M., Hrabosky, J. I., White, M. A., et al. (2008). Overvaluation of shape and weight in binge eating disorder and overweight controls: Refinement of a diagnostic construct. *Journal of Abnormal Psychology, 117*(2), 414–419. https://doi.org/10.1037/0021-843X.117.2.414.

Gross, J. J. (2002). Emotion regulation: Affective, cognitive, and social consequences. *Psychophysiology, 39*(3), 281–291.

Gross, J. J., & Thompson, R. A. (2007). Emotion regulation: Conceptual foundations. J. J. Gross (Ed.), *Handbook of emotion regulation* (pp. 3–25). The Guilford Press.

Hagan, K. E., & Walsh, B. T. (2021). State of the art: The therapeutic approaches to bulimia nervosa. *Clinical Therapeutics, 43*(1), 40–49. https://doi.org/10.1016/j.clinthera.2020.10.012.

Hale, M. A., & Clark, D. A. (2013). When good people have bad thoughts: Religiosity and the emotional regulation of guilt-inducing intrusive thoughts. *Journal of Psychology and Theology, 41*(1), 24–35.

Halmi, K. A. (2004). Obsessive-compulsive personality disorder and eating disorders. *Eating Disorders, 13*(1), 85–92.

Halmi, K. A., Sunday, S. R., Strober, M., et al. (2000). Perfectionism in anorexia nervosa: Variation by clinical subtype, obsessionality, and pathological eating behavior. *American Journal of Psychiatry, 157*, 1799–1805.

Halmi, K. A., Tozzi, F., Thornton, L. M., et al. (2005). The relation among perfectionism, obsessive-compulsive personality disorder and obsessive-compulsive disorder in individuals with eating disorders. *The International Journal of Eating Disorders, 38* (4), 371–374. https://doi.org/10.1002/eat .20190.

Hans, E., & Hiller, W. (2013). A meta-analysis of nonrandomized effectiveness studies on outpatient cognitive behavioral therapy for adult anxiety disorders. *Clinical Psychology Review, 33*(8), 954–964.

Harned, M. S., Dimeff, L. A., Woodcock, E. A., & Contreras, I. (2013). Predicting adoption of exposure therapy in a randomized controlled dissemination trial. *Journal of Anxiety Disorders, 27*(8), 754–762.

Hartmann, A., Wirth, C., & Zeeck, A. (2007). Prediction of failure of inpatient treatment of anorexia nervosa from early weight gain. *Psychotherapy Research, 17*(2), 218–229.

Hasler, G., LaSalle-Ricci, V. H., Ronquillo, J. G., et al. (2005). Obsessive-compulsive disorder symptom dimensions show specific relationships to psychiatric comorbidity. *Psychiatry Research, 135*(2), 121–132

Hatsukami, D., Mitchell, J. E., Eckert, E. D., & Pyle, R. (1986). Characteristics of patients with bulimia only, bulimia with affective disorder, and bulimia with substance abuse problems. *Addictive Behaviors, 11*(4), 399–406.

Hayes, S. C., Wilson, K. G., Gifford, E. V., Follette, V. M., & Strosahl, K. (1996). Experiential avoidance and behavioral disorders: A functional dimensional approach to diagnosis and treatment. *Journal of Consulting and Clinical Psychology, 64*(6), 1152.

Hearing, S. D. (2004). Refeeding syndrome. *BMJ, 328*(7445), 908–909.

Heatherton, T. F., & Baumeister, R. F. (1991). Binge eating as escape from self-awareness. *Psychological Bulletin, 110*(1), 86.

Herpertz-Dahlmann, B., Hebebrand, J., Müller, B., et al. (2001). Prospective 10-year follow-up in adolescent anorexia nervosa – course, outcome, psychiatric comorbidity, and psychosocial adaptation. *Journal of Child Psychology and Psychiatry and Allied Disciplines, 42*(5), 603–612.

Herzog, P., Osen, B., Stierle, C., et al. (2022). Determining prognostic variables of treatment outcome in obsessive-compulsive disorder: Effectiveness and its predictors in routine clinical care. *European Archives of Psychiatry and Clinical Neuroscience, 272*(2), 313-326

Hezel, D. M., & McNally, R. J. (2016). A theoretical review of cognitive biases and deficits in obsessive-compulsive disorder. *Biological Psychology, 121*, 221–232.

Hezel, D. M., & Simpson, H. B. (2019). Exposure and response prevention for obsessive-compulsive disorder: A review and new directions. *Indian Journal of Psychiatry, 61*(Suppl 1), S85.

Hildebrandt, T., Bacow, T., Greif, R., & Flores, A. (2014). Exposure-based family therapy (FBT-E): An open case series of a new treatment for anorexia nervosa. *Cognitive and Behavioral Practice, 21*(4), 470–484.

Hoeger, K. M., Barger, J., Carmina, E., et al. (2016). Obesity in polycystic ovary syndrome: A systematic review and meta-analysis. *Obesity Reviews, 17*(6), 473–486.

Hofer, M., & Schelling, G. (2001). Stress and eating behavior. *Physiology & Behavior, 73* (3), 435–441.

Hofmann, S. G. (2008). Cognitive processes during fear acquisition and extinction in animals and humans: Implications for exposure therapy of anxiety disorders. *Clinical Psychology Review, 28*(2), 199–210.

Hofmann, S. G., & Barlow, D. H. (2004). Social phobia (social anxiety disorder). In D. Barlow (Ed.), *Anxiety and its disorders: The nature and treatment of anxiety and panic* (2nd ed., pp. 454–476). Guilford Press.

Hofmann, S. G., & Smits, J. A. (2008). Cognitive-behavioral therapy for adult anxiety disorders: A meta-analysis of randomized placebo-controlled trials. *Journal of Clinical Psychiatry, 69*(4), 621.

Hollander, E., Friedberg, J. P., Wasserman, S., Yeh, C. C., & Iyengar, R. (2005). The case for the OCD spectrum. In J. S. Abramowitz & A. C. Houts (Eds.), *Handbook of controversial issues in obsessive-compulsive disorder* (pp. 95–118). Kluwer Academic Press.

Hrabosky, J. I., Masheb, R. M., White, M. A., & Grilo, C. M. (2007). Overvaluation of shape and weight in binge eating disorder. *Journal of Consulting and Clinical Psychology, 75*(1), 175–180. https://doi.org/10.1037/0022-006X.75.1.175.

Huang, K., & Foldi, C. J. (2022). How can animal models inform the understanding of cognitive inflexibility in patients with anorexia nervosa? *Journal of Clinical Medicine, 11*(9), 2594.

Humphreys, J. D., Clopton, J. R., & Reich, D. A. (2007). Disordered eating behavior and obsessive compulsive symptoms in college students: Cognitive and affective similarities. *Eating Disorders, 15*(3), 247–259.

Hütter, G., Ganepola, S., & Hofmann, W. K. (2009). The hematology of anorexia nervosa. *International Journal of Eating Disorders, 42*(4), 293–300.

Inozu, M., Ulukut, F. O., Ergun, G., & Alcolado, G. M. (2014). The mediating role of disgust sensitivity and thought–action fusion between religiosity and obsessive compulsive symptoms. *International Journal of Psychology, 49*(5), 334–341.

Jack, D. C. (1991). *Silencing the self: Women and depression.* Harvard University Press.

Jacoby, R. J., & Abramowitz, J. S. (2016). Inhibitory learning approaches to exposure therapy: A critical review and translation to obsessive-compulsive disorder. *Clinical Psychology Review, 49*, 28–40.

Jalal, B., McNally, R. J., Elias, J. A., Potluri, S., & Ramachandran, V. S. (2020). "Fake it till you make it"! Contaminating rubber hands ("multisensory stimulation therapy") to treat obsessive-compulsive disorder. *Frontiers in Human Neuroscience, 13*, 414.

Jansen, A., Van Den Hout, M. A., De Loof, C., Zandbergen, J., & Griez, E. (1989). A case of bulimia successfully treated by cue exposure. *Journal of Behavior Therapy and Experimental Psychiatry, 20*(4), 327–332.

Jiménez-Murcia, S., Fernández-Aranda, F., Raich, R. M., et al. (2007). Obsessive-compulsive and eating disorders: Comparison of clinical and personality features. *Psychiatry and Clinical Neurosciences, 61*(4), 385–391.

Jones, M. K., Wootton, B. M., Vaccaro, L. D., & Menzies, R. G. (2012). The impact of climate change on obsessive compulsive checking concerns. *Australian & New Zealand Journal of Psychiatry, 46*(3), 265–270.

Jovanovic, T., Norrholm, S. D., Blanding, N. Q., et al. (2010). Impaired fear inhibition is a biomarker of PTSD but not depression. *Depression and Anxiety, 27*(3), 244–251.

Kaczkurkin, A. N., & Foa, E. B. (2015). Cognitive-behavioral therapy for anxiety disorders: An update on the empirical evidence. *Dialogues in Clinical Neuroscience, 17*(3), 337.

Kamal, N., Chami, T., Andersen, A., et al. (1991). Delayed gastrointestinal transit times in anorexia nervosa and bulimia nervosa. *Gastroenterology, 101*(5), 1320–1324.

Kamphuis, J. H., & Telch, M. J. (2000). Effects of distraction and guided threat reappraisal on fear reduction during exposure-based treatments for specific fears. *Behaviour Research and Therapy, 38*(12), 1163–1181.

Karam, A. M., Fitzsimmons-Craft, E. E., Tanofsky-Kraff, M., & Wilfley, D. E. (2019). Interpersonal psychotherapy and the treatment of eating disorders. *The Psychiatric Clinics of North America, 42*(2), 205–218. https://doi.org/10.1016/j.psc.2019.01.003.

Kaye, W. H., Bulik, C. M., Thornton, L., et al. (2004). Comorbidity of anxiety disorders with anorexia and bulimia nervosa. *American Journal of Psychiatry, 161*(12), 2215–2221.

Keough, M. E., Riccardi, C. J., Timpano, K. R., Mitchell, M. A., & Schmidt, N. B. (2010). Anxiety symptomatology: The association with distress tolerance and anxiety sensitivity. *Behavior Therapy, 41*(4), 567–574.

Kerr-Gaffney, J., Harrison, A., & Tchanturia, K. (2018). Social anxiety in the eating disorders: A systematic review and meta-analysis. *Psychological Medicine, 48*(15), 2477–2491. https://doi.org/10.1017/S0033291718000752.

Keski-Rahkonen, A. (2021). Epidemiology of binge eating disorder: Prevalence, course, comorbidity, and risk factors. *Current Opinion in Psychiatry, 34*(6), 525–531. https://doi.org/10.1097/YCO .0000000000000750.

Keski-Rahkonen, A., Bulik, C. M., Pietiläinen, K. H., et al. (2007). Eating styles, overweight and obesity in young adult twins. *European Journal of Clinical Nutrition, 61*(7), 822–829.

Keski-Rahkonen, A., & Mustelin, L. (2016). Epidemiology of eating disorders in Europe: Prevalence, incidence, comorbidity, course, consequences, and risk factors. *Current Opinion in Psychiatry, 29*(6), 340–345. https://doi.org/10.1097/YCO .0000000000000278.

Keys, A., & Brožek, J. (1953). Body fat in adult man. *Physiological Reviews, 33*(3), 245–325.

Keys, A., Brožek, J., Henschel, A., Mickelsen, O., Taylor, H. L. (1950). *The biology of human starvation* (2 vols.). University of Minnesota Press.

Kimber, M., Gonzalez, A., & MacMillan, H. L. (2020). Recognizing and responding to child maltreatment: Strategies to apply when delivering family-based treatment for eating disorders. *Frontiers in Psychiatry, 11*, 678.

Kimber, M., McTavish, J. R., Couturier, J., et al. (2019). Identifying and responding to child maltreatment when delivering family-based treatment: A qualitative study. *International Journal of Eating Disorders, 52*(3), 292–298.

Kohn, M. R., & Lock, J. (2015). Family-based treatment for adolescent anorexia nervosa: Review of the literature. *Clinical Child and Family Psychology Review, 18*(2), 141–159.

Krzyszkowiak, W., Kuleta-Krzyszkowiak, M., & Krzanowska, E. (2019). Treatment of obsessive-compulsive disorders (OCD) and obsessive-compulsive-related disorders (OCRD). *Psychiatria Polska, 53*(4), 825–843.

Kvamme, J. M., Holmen, J., Wilsgaard, T., et al. (2012). Body mass index and mortality in elderly men and women: The Tromsø and HUNT studies. *Journal of Epidemiology and Community Health, 66*(7), 611–617.

Kyrios, M., Hordern, C., & Fassnacht, D. B. (2015). Predictors of response to cognitive behaviour therapy for obsessive-compulsive disorder. *International Journal of Clinical and Health Psychology, 15*(3), 181–190.

Lacey, J. H., & Moureli, E. (1986). Bulimic alcoholics: Some features of a clinical sub-group. *British Journal of Addiction, 81*(3), 389–393.

Lang, P. J., Bergen, A., & Garfield, S. (1971). *Handbook of psychotherapy and behavior change.* Wiley.

Laposa, J. M., Collimore, K. C., Hawley, L. L., & Rector, N. A. (2015). Distress tolerance in OCD and anxiety disorders, and its relationship with anxiety sensitivity and intolerance of uncertainty. *Journal of Anxiety Disorders, 33*, 8–14.

Lavender, A., Shubert, I., de Silva, P., & Treasure, J. (2006). Obsessive-compulsive beliefs and magical ideation in eating disorders. *British Journal of Clinical Psychology, 45*(3), 331–342.

Lavender, J.M., Happel, K., Anestis, M.D., Tull, M.T., & Gratz, K.L. (2015). The interactive role of distress tolerance and eating expectancies in bulimic symptoms among substance abusers. *Eating Behaviors, 16*, 88–91.

Law, C., & Boisseau, C. L. (2019). Exposure and response prevention in the treatment of obsessive-compulsive disorder: Current perspectives. *Psychology Research and Behavior Management*, 1167–1174.

Lawlor, D. A., Henly, S. J., Lingwood, B. E., & Davey Smith, G. (2008). Maternal body mass index before pregnancy and offspring body mass index in childhood: Findings from the Avon Longitudinal Study of Parents and

Children (ALSPAC). *Pediatrics, 122*(5), e907–e913.

Le Grange, D., Accurso, E. C., Lock, J., Agras, S., & Bryson, S. W. (2014). Early weight gain predicts outcome in two treatments for adolescent anorexia nervosa. *International Journal of Eating Disorders, 47*(2), 124–129.

Le Grange, D., Crosby, R. D., Rathouz, P. J., & Leventhal, B. L. (2007). A randomized controlled comparison of family-based treatment and supportive psychotherapy for adolescent bulimia nervosa. *Archives of General Psychiatry, 64*(9), 1049–1056.

Le Grange, D., Doyle, P., Crosby, R. D., & Chen, E. (2008). Early response to treatment in adolescent bulimia nervosa. *International Journal of Eating Disorders, 41*(8), 755–757.

Le Grange, D., Eckhardt, S., Dalle Grave, R., et al. (2020). Enhanced cognitive-behavior therapy and family-based treatment for adolescents with an Eating Disorder: A non-randomized effectiveness trial. *Psychological Medicine*, 1–11. Advance online publication. https://doi.org/10.1017/S0033291720004407.

Le Grange, D., Eisler, I., Dare, C., & Hodes, M. (1992). Family criticism and self-starvation: A study of expressed emotion. *Journal of Family Therapy, 14*(2), 177–192. https://doi.org/10.1046/j.1992.00451.x.

Le Grange, D., Lock, J., Agras, W. S., et al. (2012).Moderators and mediators of remission in family-based treatment and adolescent focused therapy for anorexia nervosa. *Behaviour Research and Therapy, 50* (2), 85–92.

Le Grange, D., Lock, J., Agras, W. S., Bryson, S. W., & Jo, B. (2015). Randomized clinical trial of family-based treatment and cognitive-behavioral therapy for adolescent bulimia nervosa. *Journal of the American Academy of Child and Adolescent Psychiatry, 54*(11), 886–94.e2. https://doi.org/10.1016/j.jaac.2015.08.008.

Le Grange, D., Lock, J., & Darcy, A. (2017). Family-based treatment for adolescent anorexia nervosa: Barriers to implementation in clinical practice. *The International Journal of Eating Disorders, 50*(1), 37–42.

Legenbauer, T. M. & Meule, A. (2015) Challenges in the treatment of adolescent anorexia nervosa: Is enhanced cognitive behavior therapy the answer? *Frontiers in Psychiatry 6*, 148. https://doi.org/10.3389/fpsyt.2015.00148.

Lethbridge, J., Watson, H. J., Egan, S. J., Street, H., & Nathan, P. R. (2011). The role of perfectionism, dichotomous thinking, shape and weight overvaluation, and conditional goal setting in eating disorders. *Eating Behaviors, 12*(3), 200–206.

Levinson, C. A., Brosof, L. C., Ram, S. S., et al. (2019). Obsessions are strongly related to eating disorder symptoms in anorexia nervosa and atypical anorexia nervosa. *Eating Behaviors, 34*, 101298.

Leyro, T. M., Zvolensky, M. J., & Bernstein, A. (2010). Distress tolerance and psychopathological symptoms and disorders: A review of the empirical literature among adults. *Psychological Bulletin, 136*(4), 576.

Lilenfeld, L. R., Wonderlich, S., Riso, L. P., Crosby, R., & Mitchell, J. (2006). Eating disorders and personality: A methodological and empirical review. *Clinical Psychology Review, 26*(3), 299–320.

Linardon, J., Wade, T. D., De la Piedad Garcia, X., & Brennan, L. (2017). The efficacy of cognitive-behavioral therapy for eating disorders: A systematic review and meta-analysis. *Journal of Consulting and Clinical Psychology, 85*(11), 1080.

Lindsay, M., Crino, R., & Andrews, G. (1997). Controlled trial of exposure and response prevention in obsessive-compulsive disorder. *The British Journal of Psychiatry, 171*(2), 135–139.

Linehan, M. M. (1993). *Cognitive behavioral treatment of borderline personality disorder*. Guilford Press.

Lock, J. (2005). Adjusting cognitive behavior therapy for adolescents with bulimia nervosa: Results of case series. *American Journal of Psychotherapy, 59*(3), 267–281.

Lock J. (2015). An update on evidence-based psychosocial treatments for eating disorders in children and adolescents. *Journal of Clinical Child and Adolescent Psychology, 44* (5), 707–721. https://doi.org/10.1080/15374416.2014.971458.

Lock, J., Agras, W. S., Bryson, S., & Kraemer, H. C. (2005). A comparison of short- and long-term family therapy for adolescent anorexia nervosa. *Journal of the American Academy of Child and Adolescent Psychiatry*, 44(7), 632–639. https://doi.org/10.1097/01.chi.0000161647.82775.0a.

Lock, J., Couturier, J., Bryson, S., & Agras, S. (2006). Predictors of dropout and remission in family therapy for adolescent anorexia nervosa in a randomized clinical trial. *International Journal of Eating Disorders*, 39(8), 639–647.

Lock, J., & Le Grange, D. (2001). Can family-based treatment of anorexia nervosa be manualized? *Journal of Psychotherapy Practice and Research*, 10(4), 253.

Lock, J., & Le Grange, D. (2005). Family-based treatment of eating disorders. *International Journal of Eating Disorders*, 37(S1), S64-S67.

Lock, J., & Le Grange, D. (2008). Family-based treatment of adolescent anorexia nervosa: Barriers to implementation. *Journal of the American Academy of Child and Adolescent Psychiatry*, 47(11), 1256–1263.

Lock, J., & Le Grange, D. (2013). Family-based treatment for adolescents with anorexia nervosa. *Journal of Clinical Psychology*, 69(3), 256–268.

Lock, J., & Le Grange, D. (2019). Family-based treatment: Where are we and where should we be going to improve recovery in child and adolescent eating disorders. *The International Journal of Eating Disorders*, 52(4), 481–487. https://doi.org/10.1002/eat.22980.

Lock, J., Le Grange, D., Agras, W. S., et al. (2010). A comparison of family-based treatment and adolescent-focused individual therapy for adolescents with anorexia nervosa. *Archives of Pediatrics & Adolescent Medicine*, 164(2), 188–195.

Lock, J., & Nicholls, D. (2020). Toward a greater understanding of the ways family-based treatment addresses the full range of psychopathology of adolescent anorexia nervosa. *Frontiers in Psychiatry*, 10, 968.

Loeb, K. L., & le Grange, D. (2009). Family-based treatment for adolescent eating disorders: Current status, new applications and future directions. *International Journal of Child and Adolescent Health*, 2(2), 243–254.

Lovibond, P. F., Davis, N. R., & O'Flaherty, A. S. (2000). Protection from extinction in human fear conditioning. *Behaviour Research and Therapy*, 38(10), 967–983.

Lowe, M. R., Berner, L. A., Swanson, S. A., et al. (2011). Weight suppression predicts time to remission from bulimia nervosa. *Journal of Consulting and Clinical Psychology*, 79(6), 772.

Luce, K. H., & Crowther, J. H. (1999). The reliability of the eating disorder examination: Self-report questionnaire version (EDE-Q). *International Journal of Eating Disorders*, 25(3), 349–351.

Macatee, R.J., Capron, D.W., Schmidt. N.B., & Cougle, J.R. (2013). An examination of low distress tolerance and life stressors as factors underlying obsessions. *Journal of Psychiatry Research*, 47(10), 1462–1468.

Machado, J. D. C., Suen, V. M. M., Chueire, F. B., Marchini, J. F. M., & Marchini, J. S. (2009). Refeeding syndrome, an undiagnosed and forgotten potentially fatal condition. *Case Reports*, 2009, bcr0720080521.

Madanes, C. (1981). *Strategic family therapy.* Jossey-Bass.

Madden, S., Miskovic-Wheatley, J., Clarke, S., et al. (2015). Outcomes of a rapid refeeding protocol in adolescent anorexia nervosa. *Journal of Eating Disorders*, 3(1), 1–8.

Madowitz, J., Matheson, B. E., & Liang, J. (2015). The relationship between eating disorders and sexual trauma. *Eating and Weight Disorders*, 20, 281–293.

Mandelli, L., Draghetti, S., Albert, U., De Ronchi, D., & Atti, A. R. (2020). Rates of comorbid obsessive-compulsive disorder in eating disorders: A meta-analysis of the literature. *Journal of Affective Disorders*, 277, 927–939.

Margolis, H., & McCabe, P. P. (2006). Improving self-efficacy and motivation: What to do, what to say. *Intervention in School and Clinic*, 41(4), 218–227.

Marien, W. E., Storch, E. A., Geffken, G. R., & Murphy, T. K. (2009). Intensive family-based cognitive-behavioral therapy for pediatric obsessive-compulsive disorder: Applications for treatment of medication partial- or nonresponders. *Cognitive and Behavioral Practice, 16*(3). https://doi.org/10.1016/j.cbpra.2008.12.006.

Marzola, E., Nasser, J. A., Hashim, S. A., Shih, P. A. B., & Kaye, W. H. (2013). Nutritional rehabilitation in anorexia nervosa: Review of the literature and implications for treatment. *BMC Psychiatry, 13*, 1–13.

Mathes, B. M., Day, T. N., Wilver, N. L., Redden, S. A., & Cougle, J. R. (2020). Indices of change in exposure and response prevention for contamination-based OCD. *Behaviour Research and Therapy, 133*, 103707.

McClain, Z., & Peebles, R. (2016). Body image and eating disorders among lesbian, gay, bisexual, and transgender youth. *Pediatric Clinics, 63*(6), 1079–1090.

McCubbin, R. A., & Sampson, M. J. (2006). The relationship between obsessive-compulsive symptoms and appraisals of emotional states. *Journal of Anxiety Disorders, 20*(1), 42–57.

McGuire, J. F., & Storch, E. A. (2019). An inhibitory learning approach to cognitive-behavioral therapy for children and adolescents. *Cognitive and Behavioral Practice, 26*(1), 214–224.

McIntosh, V. V. W., Carter, F. A., Bulik, C. M., et al. (2011). Five-year outcome of cognitive behavioral therapy and exposure with response prevention for bulimia nervosa. *Psychological Medicine, 41*(5), 1061–1071.

McKay, D., Sookman, D., Neziroglu, F., et al. (2015). Efficacy of cognitive-behavioral therapy for obsessive-compulsive disorder. *Psychiatry Research, 225*(3), 236–246.

McLean, P. D., Whittal, M. L., Thordarson, D. S., et al. (2001). Cognitive versus behavior therapy in the group treatment of obsessive-compulsive disorder. *Journal of Consulting and Clinical Psychology, 69*(2), 205.

Meads, C., Gold, L., & Burls, A. (2001). How effective is outpatient care compared to inpatient care for the treatment of anorexia nervosa? A systematic review. *European Eating Disorders Review: The Professional Journal of the Eating Disorders Association, 9*(4), 229–241.

Mehler, P. S., & Brown, C. (2015). Anorexia nervosa: Medical complications. *Journal of Eating Disorders, 3*, 1–8.

Meier, M., Kossakowski, J. J., Jones, P. J., et al. (2020). Obsessive-compulsive symptoms in eating disorders: A network investigation. *International Journal of Eating Disorders, 53*(3), 362–371.

Meyer, V. (1966). Modification of expectations in cases with obsessional rituals. *Behaviour Research and Therapy, 4*(4), 273–280.

Meyer, J. M., Farrell, N. R., Kemp, J. J., Blakey, S. M., & Deacon, B. J. (2014). Why do clinicians exclude anxious clients from exposure therapy? *Behaviour Research and Therapy, 54*, 49–53.

Michel, N. M., Rowa, K., Young, L., & McCabe, R. E. (2016). Emotional distress tolerance across anxiety disorders. *Journal of Anxiety Disorders, 40*, 94–103.

Middleton, R., Wheaton, M. G., Kayser, R., & Simpson, H. B. (2019). Treatment resistance in obsessive-compulsive disorder. In Y. K. Kim (Ed.), *Treatment Resistance in psychiatry: Risk factors, biology, and management* (pp. 165–177). Springer Nature Singapore Pte Ltd.

Mikhail, M. E., & Klump, K. L. (2021). A virtual issue highlighting eating disorders in people of black/African and Indigenous heritage. *International Journal of Eating Disorders, 54*(3), 459–467.

Milad, M. R., Pitman, R. K., Ellis, C. B., et al. (2009). Neurobiological basis of failure to recall extinction memory in posttraumatic stress disorder. *Biological Psychiatry, 66*(12), 1075–1082.

Miller, K. K., Grinspoon, S. K., Ciampa, J., et al. (2005). Medical findings in outpatients with anorexia nervosa. *Archives of Internal Medicine, 165*(5), 561–566.

Milos, G., Spindler, A., Ruggiero, G., Klaghofer, R., & Schnyder, U. (2002). Comorbidity of obsessive-compulsive disorders and duration of eating disorders. *International Journal of Eating Disorders, 31*(3), 284–289.

Minuchin, S. (1974). *Families and family therapy*. Tavistock Publications.

Missbach, B., Dunn, T. M., & König, J. S. (2017). We need new tools to assess orthorexia nervosa. A commentary on "prevalence of orthorexia nervosa among college students based on Bratman's test and associated tendencies." *Appetite, 108*(1), 521–524.

Mitchell, J. E., Pyle, R. L., Pomeroy, C., et al. (1993). Cognitive-behavioral group psychotherapy of bulimia nervosa: Importance of logistical variables. *The International journal of Eating Disorders, 14* (3), 277–287. https://doi.org/10.1002/1098-1 08x(199311)14:3<277::aid-eat2260140306>3.0.co;2-8.

Mitchell, K. S., Scioli, E. R., Galovski, T., Belfer, P. L., & Cooper, Z. (2021). Posttraumatic stress disorder and eating disorders: Maintaining mechanisms and treatment targets. *Eating Disorders, 29*(3), 292–306.

Moscovitch, D. A. (2009). What is the core fear in social phobia? A new model to facilitate individualized case conceptualization and treatment. *Cognitive and Behavioral Practice, 16*(2), 123–134.

Mulkens, S., de Vos, C., de Graaff, A., & Waller, G. (2018). To deliver or not to deliver cognitive behavioral therapy for eating disorders: Replication and extension of our understanding of why therapists fail to do what they should do. *Behaviour Research and Therapy, 106*, 57–63.

Murphy, R., Cooper, Z., Hollon, S. D., & Fairburn, C. G. (2009). How do psychological treatments work? Investigating mediators of change. *Behaviour Research and Therapy, 47* (1), 1–5.

Murray, K., Jassi, A., Mataix-Cols, D., Barrow, F., & Krebs, G. (2015). Outcomes of cognitive behaviour therapy for obsessive-compulsive disorder in young people with and without autism spectrum disorders: A case controlled study. *Psychiatry Research, 228*(1), 8–13.

Naragon-Gainey, K., McMahon, T. P., & Chacko, T. P. (2017). The structure of common emotion regulation strategies: A meta-analytic examination. *Psychological Bulletin, 143*(4), 384.

Neziroglu, F., & Sandler, J. (2009). The relationship between eating disorders and OCD part of the spectrum. *OCD Newsletter 2009, 23*(3).

NICE. (2020). *Recommendations: Eating disorders: Recognition and treatment: Guidance*. National Institute for Health and Care Excellence (NICE). December 16, 2020. Retrieved January 22, 2023, from www .nice.org.uk/guidance/ng69/chapter/Recom mendations#treating-bulimia-nervosa.

Nicely, T. A., Lane-Loney, S., Masciulli, E., Hollenbeak, C. S., & Ornstein, R. M. (2014). Prevalence and characteristics of avoidant/ restrictive food intake disorder in a cohort of young patients in day treatment for eating disorders. *Journal of Eating Disorders, 2*(1), 21. https://doi.org/10.1186/s40337-014-0021-3.

Nisbett, R. E. (1972). Hunger, obesity, and the ventromedial hypothalamus. *Psychological Review, 79*(6), 433.

Nock, M. K., & Mendes, W. B. (2008). Physiological arousal, distress tolerance, and social problem-solving deficits among adolescent self-injurers. *Journal of Consulting and Clinical Psychology, 76*(1), 28.

Norr, A. M., Oglesby, M. E., Capron, D. W., et al. (2013). Evaluating the unique contribution of intolerance of uncertainty relative to other cognitive vulnerability factors in anxiety psychopathology. *Journal of Affective Disorders, 151*(1), 136–142.

Norton, P. J., & Price, E. C. (2007). A meta-analytic review of adult cognitive-behavioral treatment outcome across the anxiety disorders. *Journal of Nervous and Mental Disease, 195*(6), 521–531.

Obsessive Compulsive Cognitions Working Group. (1997). Cognitive assessment of obsessive-compulsive disorder. *Behaviour Research and Therapy, 35*(7), 667–681.

Olatunji, B. O., Cisler, J. M., & Deacon, B. J. (2010). Efficacy of cognitive behavioral therapy for anxiety disorders: A review of meta-analytic findings. *Psychiatric Clinics, 33* (3), 557–577.

Olatunji, B. O., Davis, M. L., Powers, M. B., & Smits, J. A. (2013). Cognitive-behavioral therapy for obsessive-compulsive disorder: A meta-analysis of treatment outcome and moderators. *Journal of Psychiatric Research*, *47*(1), 33–41.

Olmsted, M. P., Davis, R., Rockert, W., et al. (1991). Efficacy of a brief group psychoeducational intervention for bulimia nervosa. *Behaviour Research and Therapy*, *29*(1), 71–83.

Ougrin, D. (2011). Efficacy of exposure versus cognitive therapy in anxiety disorders: Systematic review and meta-analysis. *BMC Psychiatry*, *11*(1), 1–13.

Pallister, E., & Waller, G. (2008). Anxiety in the eating disorders: Understanding the overlap. *Clinical Psychology Review*, *28*(3), 366–386.

Papadopoulos, F. C., Ekbom, A., Brandt, L., & Ekselius, L. (2009). Excess mortality, causes of death and prognostic factors in anorexia nervosa. *The British Journal of Psychiatry*, *194*(1), 10–17.

Parker, Z. J., & Waller, G. (2017). Development and validation of the Negative Attitudes towards CBT Scale. *Behavioural and Cognitive Psychotherapy*, *45*(6), 629–646.

Parker, Z. J., Waller, G., Gonzalez Salas Duhne, P., & Dawson, J. (2018). The role of exposure in treatment of anxiety disorders: A meta-analysis. *International Journal of Psychology and Psychological Therapy*, *18*(1), 111–141.

Parrish, C. L., Radomsky, A. S., & Dugas, M. J. (2008). Anxiety-control strategies: Is there room for neutralization in successful exposure treatment? *Clinical Psychology Review*, *28*(8), 1400–1412.

Passmore, R., Melklejohn, A. P., Dewar, A. D., & Thow, R. K. (1955). An analysis of the gain in weight of overfed thin young men. *British Journal of Nutrition*, *9*(1), 27–37.

Pato, M. T., Zohar-Kadouch, R., Zohar, J., & Murphy, D. L. (1988). Return of symptoms after discontinuation of clomipramine in patients with obsessive-compulsive disorder. *The American Journal of Psychiatry*, *145*(12), 1521–1525.

Peebles, R., Hardy, K. K., Wilson, J. L., & Lock, J. D. (2010). Are diagnostic criteria for eating disorders markers of medical severity? *Pediatrics*, *125*(5), e1193–e1201.

Peebles, R., Lesser, A., Park, C. C., et al. (2017). Outcomes of an inpatient medical nutritional rehabilitation protocol in children and adolescents with eating disorders. *Journal of Eating Disorders*, *5*(1), 1–14.

Peebles, R., & Sieke, E. H. (2019). Medical complications of eating disorders in youth. *Child and Adolescent Psychiatric Clinics*, *28*(4), 593–615.

Pellizzer, M. L., Waller, G., & Wade, T. D. (2019). A pragmatic effectiveness study of 10-session cognitive behavioural therapy (CBT-T) for eating disorders: Targeting barriers to treatment provision. *European Eating Disorders Review*, *27*(5), 557–570.

Peterson, C. M., Davis-Becker, K., & Fischer, S. (2014). Interactive role of depression, distress tolerance and negative urgency on non-suicidal self-injury. *Personality and Mental Health*, *8*(2), 151–160.

Phillips, K. A., & Diedrichs, P. C. (2015). Men, muscles, and moods: A review of the relationships between appearance concerns, body image, and depression. *Body Image*, *12*, 44–53.

Phillips, K. A., Hart, A. S., & Menard, W. (2014). Psychometric evaluation of the Yale–Brown obsessive-compulsive scale modified for body dysmorphic disorder (BDD-YBOCS). *Journal of Obsessive-Compulsive and Related Disorders*, *3*(3), 205–208.

Pietrefesa, A. S., & Coles, M. E. (2008). Moving beyond an exclusive focus on harm avoidance in obsessive compulsive disorder: Considering the role of incompleteness. *Behavior Therapy*, *39*(3), 224–231.

Pinel, J. P., Assanand, S., & Lehman, D. R. (2000). Hunger, eating, and ill health. *American Psychologist*, *55*(10), 1105.

Pinto, A., Liebowitz, M. R., Foa, E. B., & Simpson, H. B. (2011). Obsessive compulsive personality disorder as a predictor of exposure and ritual prevention outcome for obsessive compulsive disorder. *Behaviour Research and Therapy*, *49*(8), 453–458.

Pollack, L. O., & Forbush, K. T. (2013). Why do eating disorders and obsessive-compulsive disorder co-occur? *Eating Behaviors, 14*(2), 211–215.

Pollice, C., Kaye, W. H., Greeno, C. G., & Weltzin, T. E. (1997). Relationship of depression, anxiety, and obsessionality to state of illness in anorexia nervosa. *The International journal of Eating Disorders, 21* (4), 367–376. https://doi.org/10.1002/(sici)1 098-108x(1997)21:4<367::aid-eat10>3.0. co;2-w.

Poulsen, S., Lunn, S., Daniel, S. I., Folke, S., et al. (2014). A randomized controlled trial of psychoanalytic psychotherapy or cognitive-behavioral therapy for bulimia nervosa. *The American Journal of Psychiatry, 171*(1), 109–116. https://doi.org/10.1176/app i.ajp.2013.12121511.

Powers, M. B., Smits, J. A., & Telch, M. J. (2004). Disentangling the effects of safety-behavior utilization and safety-behavior availability during exposure-based treatment: A placebo-controlled trial. *Journal of Consulting and Clinical Psychology, 72*(3), 448.

Pretorius, N., Dimmer, M., Power, E., et al. (2012). Evaluation of a cognitive remediation therapy group for adolescents with anorexia nervosa: Pilot study. *European Eating Disorders Review, 20*(4), 321–325.

Puhl, R., Peterson, J. L., & Luedicke, J. (2013). Fighting obesity or obese persons? Public perceptions of obesity-related health messages. *International Journal of Obesity, 37*(6), 774–782.

Quirk, G. J. (2002). Memory for extinction of conditioned fear is long-lasting and persists following spontaneous recovery. *Learning & Memory, 9*(6), 402–407.

Rachman S. (1993). Obsessions, responsibility and guilt. *Behaviour Research and Therapy, 31*(2), 149–154. https://doi.org/10.1016/0005-7967(93)90066-4.

Rachman S. (1997). A cognitive theory of obsessions. *Behaviour Research and Therapy, 35*(9), 793–802. https://doi.org/10.1016/s000 5-7967(97)00040-5.

Rachman, S. (2002). A cognitive theory of compulsive checking. *Behaviour Research and Therapy, 40*(6), 625–639.

Rachman, S., & de Silva, P. (1978). Abnormal and normal obsessions. *Behaviour Research and Therapy, 16*(4), 233–248. https://doi.org /10.1016/0005-7967(78)90022-0.

Rachman, S. J., & Hodgson, R. J. (1980). *Obsessions and compulsions.* Prentice Hall.

Rachman, S., Hodgson, R., & Marks, I. M. (1971). The treatment of chronic obsessive-compulsive neurosis. *Behaviour Research and Therapy, 9*(3), 237–247.

Rachman, S., & Shafran, R. (1999). Cognitive distortions: Thought–action fusion. *Clinical Psychology & Psychotherapy: An International Journal of Theory & Practice, 6* (2), 80–85.

Racine, S. E., VanHuysse, J. L., Keel, P. K., et al. (2017). Eating disorder-specific risk factors moderate the relationship between negative urgency and binge eating: A behavioral genetic investigation. *Journal of Abnormal Psychology, 126*(5), 481–494.

Raines, A. M., Oglesby, M. E., Allan, N. P., et al. (2018). Examining the role of sex differences in obsessive-compulsive symptom dimensions. *Psychiatry Research, 259,* 265–269.

Raney, T. J., Thornton, L. M., Berrettini, W., et al. (2008). Influence of overanxious disorder of childhood on the expression of anorexia nervosa. *The International Journal of Eating Disorders, 41*(4), 326–332. https:// doi.org/10.1002/eat.20508.

Rasmussen, K. M., & Yaktine, A. L. (2009). Weight gain during pregnancy: Reexamining the guidelines.

Rasmussen, S. A., & Eisen, J. L. (1992). The epidemiology and differential diagnosis of obsessive-compulsive disorder. *Zwangsstörungen/obsessive-compulsive disorders,* 1–14.

Rauch, S., & Foa, E. (2006). Emotional processing theory (EPT) and exposure therapy for PTSD. *Journal of Contemporary Psychotherapy, 36,* 61–65.

Reas, D. L., & Grilo, C. M. (2015). Pharmacological treatment of binge eating disorder: Update review and synthesis. *Expert Opinion on Pharmacotherapy, 16*(10),

1463–1478. https://doi.org/10.1517/14656566.2015.1053465.

Reid, J. E., Laws, K. R., Drummond, L., et al. (2021). Cognitive behavioural therapy with exposure and response prevention in the treatment of obsessive-compulsive disorder: A systematic review and meta-analysis of randomised controlled trials. *Comprehensive Psychiatry, 106*, 152223.

Reiser, L. W. (1990). The oral triad and the bulimic quintet: Understanding the bulimic episode. *International Review of Psycho-Analysis, 17*, 239–248.

Reisner, S. L., White Hughto, J. M., Pachankis, J. E., & Dunham, E. E. (2015). Body dissatisfaction, disordered eating, and weight cycling among transgender and gender nonconforming adults. *Psychology of Sexual Orientation and Gender Diversity, 2* (4), 312–323.

Reiss, S., Peterson, R. A., Gursky, D. M., & McNally, R. J. (1986). Anxiety sensitivity, anxiety frequency and the prediction of fearfulness. *Behaviour Research and Therapy, 24*(1), 1–8.

Rescorla, R. A. (2006). Deepened extinction from compound stimulus presentation. *Journal of Experimental Psychology: Animal Behavior Processes, 32*(2), 135–144. https://doi.org/10.1037/0097-7403.32.2.135.

Resick, P. A., Nishith, P., Weaver, T. L., Astin, M. C., & Feuer, C. A. (2002). A comparison of cognitive-processing therapy with prolonged exposure and a waiting condition for the treatment of chronic posttraumatic stress disorder in female rape victims. *Journal of Consulting and Clinical Psychology, 70*(4), 867.

Reuven, O., Liberman, N., & Dar, R. (2014). The effect of physical cleaning on threatened morality in individuals with obsessive-compulsive disorder. *Clinical Psychological Science, 2*(2), 224–229.

Richard, D. C., & Gloster, A. T. (2007). Exposure therapy has a public relations problem: A dearth of litigation amid a wealth of concern. In *Handbook of exposure therapies* (pp. 409–425). Academic Press.

Robb, C. E., De Jager, C. A., Ahmadi-Abhari, S., et al. (2020). Associations of social isolation with anxiety and depression during the early COVID-19 pandemic: A survey of older adults in London, UK. *Frontiers in Psychiatry, 11*, 591120.

Roberts, M. E. (2006). Disordered eating and obsessive-compulsive symptoms in a sub-clinical student population. *New Zealand Journal of Psychiatry, 35*, 45–54.

Rodriguez, B. I., & Craske, M. G. (1993). The effects of distraction during exposure to phobic stimuli. *Behaviour Research and Therapy, 31*(6), 549–558.

Roelofs, J., Nederkoorn, C., Jansen, A., & van der Lely, A.-J. (2008). Effects of stress on eating behavior: Conclusions from experimental studies. *Appetite, 51*(2), 556–561.

Roncero, M., Perpiñá, C., & García-Soriano, G. (2011). Study of obsessive compulsive beliefs: Relationship with eating disorders. *Behavioural and Cognitive Psychotherapy, 39* (4), 457–470. https://doi.org/10.1017/S1352465811000099.

Root, M. P., & Fallon, P. (1989). Treating the victimized bulimic: The functions of binge-purge behavior. *Journal of Interpersonal Violence, 4*(1), 90–100.

Rowe, M. K., & Craske, M. G. (1998). Effects of varied-stimulus exposure training on fear reduction and return of fear. *Behaviour Research and Therapy, 36*(7–8), 719–734.

Rudman, L. A., & Phelan, J. E. (2008). Backlash effects for disconfirming gender stereotypes in organizations. *Research in Organizational Behavior, 28*, 61–79.

Russell, G. F. M., & Mezey, A. G. (1962). An analysis of weight gain in patients with anorexia nervosa treated with high calorie diets. *Clinical Science, 23*, 449–461.

Rytwinski, N. K. (2012). Review of Jonathan S. Abramowitz, Brett J. Deacon, Stephen PH Whiteside: *Exposure Therapy for Anxiety: Principles and Practice: The Guilford Press, New York, 2011,* 398 pp, $45 (44 Figures; 14 Tables). *Journal of Contemporary Psychotherapy, 42*, 123–124.

Safer, D. L., Robinson, A. H., & Jo, B. (2010). Outcome from a randomized controlled trial of group therapy for binge eating disorder: Comparing dialectical behavior therapy adapted for binge eating to an active comparison group therapy. *Behavior Therapy, 41*(1), 106–120. https://doi.org/10.1016/j.beth.2009.01.006.

Salkovskis, P. M. (1985). Obsessional-compulsive problems: A cognitive-behavioural analysis. *Behaviour Research and Therapy, 23*(5), 571–583.

Salkovskis, P. M. (1991). The importance of behavior in the maintenance of anxiety and panic: A cognitive account. *Behavioral Psychotherapy Special Issue: The Hanging Face of Behavioral Psychotherapy, 19*, 6–19.

Sauro, C. L., Ravaldi, C., Cabras, P. L., Faravelli, C., & Ricca, V. (2008). Stress, hypothalamic-pituitary-adrenal axis and eating disorders. *Neuropsychobiology, 57*(3), 95–115.

Schebendach, J. E., Mayer, L. E., Devlin, M. J., et al. (2008). Dietary energy density and diet variety as predictors of outcome in anorexia nervosa. *The American Journal of Clinical Nutrition, 87*(4), 810–816.

Schulze, D., Kathmann, N., & Reuter, B. (2018). Getting it just right: A reevaluation of OCD symptom dimensions integrating traditional and Bayesian approaches. *Journal of Anxiety Disorders, 56*, 63–73.

Schumacher, S., Gaudlitz, K., Plag, J., et al. (2014). Who is stressed? A pilot study of salivary cortisol and alpha-amylase concentrations in agoraphobic patients and their novice therapists undergoing in vivo exposure. *Psychoneuroendocrinology, 49*, 280–289.

Schumacher, S., Miller, R., Fehm, L., et al. (2015). Therapists' and patients' stress responses during graduated versus flooding in vivo exposure in the treatment of specific phobia: A preliminary observational study. *Psychiatry Research, 230*(2), 668–675.

Scolnick, B., Zupec-Kania, B., Calabrese, L., Aoki, C., & Hildebrandt, T. (2020). Remission from chronic anorexia nervosa with ketogenic diet and ketamine: Case report. *Psychiatry, 30, 11*, 763. https://doi.org/10.3389/fpsyt.2020.00763.

Selvini-Palazzoli, M. (1974). *Self-starvation: From the intrapsychic to the transpersonal approach to anorexia nervosa.* Chaucer.

Semiz, U. B., Inanc, L., & Bezgin, C. H. (2014). Are trauma and dissociation related to treatment resistance in patients with obsessive-compulsive disorder? *Social Psychiatry and Psychiatric Epidemiology, 49*, 1287–1296.

Shafran, R. (2002). Eating disorders and obsessive compulsive disorder. In R. O. Frost & G. Steketee (Eds.), *Cognitive approaches to obsessions and compulsions* (pp. 215–231). Pergamon.

Shafran, R., Cooper, Z., & Fairburn, C. G. (2002). Clinical perfectionism: A cognitive-behavioural analysis. *Behaviour Research and Therapy, 40*(7), 773–791. https://doi.org/10.1016/s0005-7967(01)00059-6.

Shafran, R., Fairburn, C. G., Robinson, P., & Lask, B. (2004). Body checking and its avoidance in eating disorders. *The International Journal of Eating Disorders, 35*(1), 93–101. https://doi.org/10.1002/eat.10228.

Shafran, R., & Robinson, P. (2004). Thought-shape fusion in eating disorders. *British Journal of Clinical Psychology, 43*(4), 399–408.

Shafran, R., Teachman, B. A., Kerry, S., & Rachman, S. (1999). A cognitive distortion associated with eating disorders: Thought-shape fusion. *British Journal of Clinical Psychology, 38*(2), 167–179.

Shapiro, J. R., Berkman, N. D., Brownley, K. A., et al. (2007). Bulimia nervosa treatment: A systematic review of randomized controlled trials. *The International Journal of Eating Disorders, 40*(4), 321–336. https://doi.org/10.1002/eat.20372.

Sica, C., Novara, C., & Sanavio, E. (2002). Religiousness and obsessive-compulsive cognitions and symptoms in an Italian population. *Behaviour Research and Therapy, 40*(7), 813–823.

Silberg, J. L., & Bulik, C. M. (2005). The developmental association between eating disorders symptoms and symptoms of depression and anxiety in juvenile twin girls. *Journal of Child Psychology and Psychiatry, 46*(12), 1317–1326.

Simons, J.S. & Gaher, R.M. (2005). The distress tolerance scale: Development and validation of a self-report measure. *Motivation and Emotion*, 29(2), 83–102.

Simpson, H. B., Marcus, S. M., Zuckoff, A., Franklin, M., & Foa, E. B. (2012). Patient adherence to cognitive-behavioral therapy predicts long-term outcome in obsessive-compulsive disorder. *Journal of Clinical Psychiatry*, 73(9), 13941.

Simpson, H. B., Wetterneck, C. T., Cahill, S. P., et al. (2013). Treatment of obsessive-compulsive disorder complicated by comorbid eating disorders. *Cognitive Behaviour Therapy*, 42(1), 64–76. https://doi.org/10.1080/16506073.2012.751124.

Simpson, H. B., Liebowitz, M. R., Foa, E. B., et al. (2004). Post-treatment effects of exposure therapy and clomipramine in obsessive-compulsive disorder. *Depression and Anxiety*, 19(4), 225–233.

Skapinakis, P., Caldwell, D., Hollingworth, W., et al. (2016). A systematic review of the clinical effectiveness and cost-effectiveness of pharmacological and psychological interventions for the management of obsessive-compulsive disorder in children/adolescents and adults. *Health Technology Assessment*, 20(43), 1–392. https://doi.org/10.3310/hta20430.

Skowrońska, A., Sójta, K., & Strzelecki, D. (2019). Refeeding syndrome as treatment complication of anorexia nervosa. *Psychiatria Polska*, 53(5), 1113–1123.

Smink, F. R., Van Hoeken, D., & Hoek, H. W. (2012). Epidemiology of eating disorders: incidence, prevalence and mortality rates. *Current Psychiatry Reports*, 14(4), 406–414.

Soreni, N., Streiner, D., McCabe, R., et al. (2014). Dimensions of perfectionism in children and adolescents with obsessive-compulsive disorder. *Journal of the Canadian Academy of Child and Adolescent Psychiatry*, 23(2), 136.

Speranza, M., Corcos, M., Godart, N., et al. (2001). Obsessive compulsive disorders in eating disorders. *Eating Behaviors*, 2(3), 193–207.

Spettigue, W., Norris, M.L. (2019). Understanding and treating avoidant restrictive food intake disorder in children and adolescents. *Psychiatric Times*. Retrieved: www.psychiatrictimes.com/view/understand

ing-and-treating-avoidant-restrictive-food-intake-disorder-children-and-adolescents.

Steinglass, J., Albano, A. M., Simpson, H. B., et al. (2012). Fear of food as a treatment target: Exposure and response prevention for anorexia nervosa in an open series. *International Journal of Eating Disorders*, 45(4), 615–621.

Steinglass, J. E., Eisen, J. L., Attia, E., Mayer, L., & Walsh, B. T. (2007). Is anorexia nervosa a delusional disorder? An assessment of eating beliefs in anorexia nervosa. *Journal of Psychiatric Practice*, 13(2), 65–71.

Steinglass, J. E., Sysko, R., Glasofer, D., et al. (2011). Rationale for the application of exposure and response prevention to the treatment of anorexia nervosa. *International Journal of Eating Disorders*, 44(2), 134–141. https://doi.org/10.1002/eat.20784.

Steinhausen, H. C. (2009). Outcome of eating disorders. *Child and Adolescent Psychiatric Clinics of North America*, 18(1), 225–242.

Steketee, G. (1993). Social support and treatment outcome of obsessive compulsive disorder at 9-month follow-up. *Behavioural and Cognitive Psychotherapy*, 21(2), 81–95.

Steketee, G., Siev, J., Fama, J. M., et al. (2011). Predictors of treatment outcome in modular cognitive therapy for obsessive-compulsive disorder. *Depression and Anxiety*, 28(4), 333–341.

Stice, E. (2002). Risk and maintenance factors for eating pathology: A meta-analytic review. *Psychological Bulletin*, 128(5), 825–848. https://doi.org/10.1037/0033-2909.128.5.825.

Sternheim, L., Startup, H., & Schmidt, U. (2011). An experimental exploration of behavioral and cognitive–emotional aspects of intolerance of uncertainty in eating disorder patients. *Journal of Anxiety Disorders*, 25(6), 806–812.

Storch, E. A., Abramowitz, J. S., & Keeley, M. (2009). Correlates and mediators of functional disability in obsessive-compulsive disorder. *Depression and Anxiety*, 26(9), 806–813.

Storch, E. A., Geffken, G. R., Merlo, L. J., et al. (2007). Family-based cognitive-behavioral therapy for pediatric obsessive-compulsive disorder: Comparison of intensive and weekly approaches. *Journal of the American Academy of Child & Adolescent Psychiatry, 46* (4), 469–478.

Storch, E. A., Lehmkuhl, H. D., Ricketts, E., et al. (2010). An open trial of intensive family based cognitive-behavioral therapy in youth with obsessive-compulsive disorder who are medication partial responders or nonresponders. *Journal of Clinical Child & Adolescent Psychology, 39*(2), 260–268.

Storch, E. A., Merlo, L. J., Larson, M. J., et al. (2008). Symptom dimensions and cognitive-behavioural therapy outcome for pediatric obsessive-compulsive disorder. *Acta Psychiatrica Scandinavica, 117*(1), 67–75.

Stoll, L. C., & Egner, J. (2021). We must do better: Ableism and fatphobia in sociology. *Sociology Compass, 15*(4), e12869.

Strober, M. (2004) Pathologic fear conditioning and anorexia nervosa: On the search for novel paradigms. *International Journal of Eating Disorders, 35*, 504–508.

Strober, M., Freeman, R., Lampert, C., & Diamond, J. (2007). The association of anxiety disorders and obsessive compulsive personality disorder with anorexia nervosa: Evidence from a family study with discussion of nosological and neurodevelopmental implications. *International Journal of Eating Disorders, 40*(S3), S46-S51.

Strumia, R., Borghi, A., Colombo, E., Manzato, E., & Gualandi, M. (2005). Low prevalence of twisted hair in anorexia nervosa. *Clinical and Experimental Dermatology, 30*(4), 349–350.

Summerfeldt, L. J. (2004). Understanding and treating incompleteness in obsessive-compulsive disorder. *Journal of Clinical Psychology, 60*(11), 1155–1168.

Summerfeldt, L. J., Gilbert, S. J., & Reynolds, M. (2015). Incompleteness, aesthetic sensitivity, and the obsessive-compulsive need for symmetry. *Journal of Behavior Therapy and Experimental Psychiatry, 49*, 141–149.

Sunday, S. R., Halmi, K. A., & Einhorn, A. (1995). The Yale-Brown-Cornell Eating Disorder Scale: A new scale to assess eating disorder symptomatology. *The International Journal of Eating Disorders, 18*(3), 237–245.

https://doi.org/10.1002/1098-108x(199511)1 8:3<237::aid-eat2260180305>3.0.co;2-1.

Swinbourne, J. M., & Touyz, S. W. (2007). The co-morbidity of eating disorders and anxiety disorders: A review. *European Eating Disorders Review: The Professional Journal of the Eating Disorders Association, 15*(4), 253–274. https://doi.org/10.1002/erv.784.

Sysko, R., & Walsh, B. T. (2008). A critical evaluation of the efficacy of self-help interventions for the treatment of bulimia nervosa and binge-eating disorder. *The International Journal of Eating Disorders, 41* (2), 97–112. https://doi.org/10.1002/eat .20475.

Tek, C., & Ulug, B. (2001). Religiosity and religious obsessions in obsessive-compulsive disorder. *Psychiatry Research, 104*(2), 99–108.

Telch, M. J., Valentiner, D. P., Ilai, D., et al. (2004). Fear activation and distraction during the emotional processing of claustrophobic fear. *Journal of Behavior Therapy and Experimental Psychiatry, 35*(3), 219–232.

Thomas, J. J., Becker, K. R., Breithaupt, L., et al. (2021). Cognitive-behavioral therapy for adults with avoidant/restrictive food intake disorder. *Journal of Behavioral and Cognitive Therapy, 31*(1), 47–55.

Thomas, J. J., Becker, K. R., Kuhnle, M. C., et al. (2020). Cognitive-behavioral therapy for avoidant/restrictive food intake disorder: Feasibility, acceptability, and proof of concept for children and adolescents. *International Journal of Eating Disorders, 53* (10), 1636–1646.

Thomas, J. J., Brigham, K. S., Sally, S. T., Hazen, E. P., & Eddy, K. T. (2017). Case 18–2017: An 11-year-old girl with difficulty eating after a choking incident. *New England Journal of Medicine, 376*(24), 2377–2386.

Thomas, J. J., & Eddy, K. T. (2018). *Cognitive-behavioral therapy for avoidant/ restrictive food intake disorder: Children, adolescents, and adults.* Cambridge University Press.

Thomas, J. J., Wons, O. B., & Eddy, K. T. (2018). Cognitive-behavioral treatment of avoidant/ restrictive food intake disorder. *Current*

Opinion in Psychiatry, 31(6), 425–430. https://doi.org/10.1097/YCO.0000000000000454.

Thompson, J. K., & Heinberg, L. J. (1999). The media's influence on body image disturbance and eating disorders: We've reviled them, now can we rehabilitate them? Journal of Social Issues, 55(2), 339–353.

Tiggemann, M., Slater, A., & Slater, S. (2017). NetGirls: The Internet, Facebook, and the body image concerns of adolescent girls. Body Image, 21, 65–70.

Tobin, D. L., Banker, J. D., Weisberg, L., & Bowers, W. (2007). I know what you did last summer (and it was not CBT): A factor analytic model of international psychotherapeutic practice in the eating disorders. International Journal of Eating Disorders, 40(8), 754–757.

Tolin, D. F. (2009). Alphabet Soup: ERP, CT, and ACT for OCD. Cognitive and Behavioral Practice, 16(1), 40–48.

Tolin, D. F., Abramowitz, J. S., Brigidi, B. D., & Foa, E. B. (2003). Intolerance of uncertainty in obsessive-compulsive disorder. Journal of Anxiety Disorders, 17(2), 233–242.

Tolin, D. F., Gilliam, C., Wootton, B. M., et al. (2018). Psychometric properties of a structured diagnostic interview for DSM-5 anxiety, mood, and obsessive-compulsive and related disorders. Assessment, 25 (1), 3–13.

Treasure, J., & Russell, G. (2011). The case for early intervention in anorexia nervosa: Theoretical exploration of maintaining factors. The British Journal of Psychiatry, 199 (1), 5–7.

Trentowska, M., Svaldi, J., & Tuschen-Caffier, B. (2014). Efficacy of body exposure as treatment component for patients with eating disorders. Journal of Behavior Therapy and Experimental Psychiatry, 45(1), 178–185.

Trottier, K., & MacDonald, D. E. (2017). Update on psychological trauma, other severe adverse experiences and eating disorders: State of the research and future research directions. Current Psychiatry Reports, 19, 1–9.

Tundo, A., & Necci, R. (2016). Cognitive-behavioural therapy for obsessive-compulsive disorder co-occurring with psychosis: Systematic review of evidence. World Journal of Psychiatry, 6 (4), 449.

Tyagi, H., Patel, R., Rughooputh, F., et al. (2015). Comparative prevalence of eating disorders in obsessive-compulsive disorder and other anxiety disorders. Psychiatry Journal, 2015, 1–6.

Uri, R. C., Wu, Y. K., Baker, J. H., & Munn-Chernoff, M. A. (2021). Eating disorder symptoms in Asian American college students. Eating Behaviors, 40, 101458.

Vall, E., & Wade, T. D. (2015). Predictors of treatment outcome in individuals with eating disorders: A systematic review and meta-analysis. The International Journal of Eating Disorders, 48(7), 946–971. https://doi.org/10.1002/eat.22411.

van Balkom, A. J., van Oppen, P., Vermeulen, A., & Blom, M. B. (2008). Exposure therapy for anxiety disorders: A meta-analysis. Journal of Consulting and Clinical Psychology, 76(6), 1038–1047.

Van Eck, K., Warren, P., & Flory, K. (2017). A variable-centered and person-centered evaluation of emotion regulation and distress tolerance: Links to emotional and behavioral concerns. Journal of Youth and Adolescence, 46(1), 136–150.

Van Eeden, A. E., van Hoeken, D., & Hoek, H. W. (2021). Incidence, prevalence and mortality of anorexia nervosa and bulimia nervosa. Current Opinion in Psychiatry, 34(6), 515.

Van Oppen, P., Hoekstra, R. J., & Emmelkamp, P. M. (1995). The structure of obsessive-compulsive symptoms. Behaviour Research and Therapy, 33(1), 15–23.

Vanzhula, I. A., Kinkel-Ram, S. S., & Levinson, C. A. (2021). Perfectionism and difficulty controlling thoughts bridge eating disorder and obsessive-compulsive disorder symptoms: A network analysis. Journal of Affective Disorders, 283, 302–309.

Veale, D. (2002). Over-valued ideas: A conceptual analysis. Behaviour Research and Therapy, 40(4), 383–400.

Vervaet, M., Van Heeringen, C., & Audenaert, K. (2004). Personality-related characteristics in restricting versus bingeing and purging eating disordered patients. *Comprehensive Psychiatry, 45*(1), 37–43.

Waller, G. (2009). Evidence-based treatment and therapist drift. *Behaviour Research and Therapy, 47*(2), 119–127.

Waller, G. (2016). Treatment protocols for eating disorders: clinicians' attitudes, concerns, adherence and difficulties delivering evidence-based psychological interventions. *Current Psychiatry Reports, 18*, 1–8.

Waller, G., & Mountford, V. A. (2015). Weighing patients within cognitive-behavioural therapy for eating disorders: How, when and why. *Behaviour Research and Therapy, 70*, 1–10.

Waller, G., & Raykos, B. (2019). Behavioral interventions in the treatment of eating disorders. *Psychiatric Clinics, 42*(2), 181–191.

Waller, G., Gray, E., Hinrichsen, H., et al. (2014). Cognitive-behavioral therapy for bulimia nervosa and atypical bulimic nervosa: Effectiveness in clinical settings. *International Journal of Eating Disorders, 47*(1), 13–17.

Waller, G., Stringer, H., & Meyer, C. (2012). What cognitive behavioral techniques do therapists report using when delivering cognitive behavioral therapy for the eating disorders? *Journal of Consulting and Clinical Psychology, 80*(1), 171–175. https://doi.org/10.1037/a0026559.

Waller, G., Tatham, M., Turner, H., et al. (2018). A 10-session cognitive-behavioral therapy (CBT-T) for eating disorders: Outcomes from a case series of non underweight adult patients. *International Journal of Eating Disorders, 51*(3), 262–269.

Waller, G., Turner, H. M., Tatham, M., Mountford, V. A., & Wade, T. D. (2018). *Brief cognitive behavioural therapy for non-underweight patients: CBT-T for eating disorders*. Routledge.

Walker, J., Roberts, S. L., Halmi, K. A., & Goldberg, S. C. (1979). Caloric requirements for weight gain in anorexia nervosa. *The American Journal of Clinical Nutrition, 32*(7), 1396–1400.

Walsh, B. T., Wilson, G. T., Loeb, K. L., et al. (1997). Medication and psychotherapy in the treatment of bulimia nervosa. *The American Journal of Psychiatry, 154*(4), 523–531. https://doi.org/10.1176/ajp.154.4.523.

Wang, G. J., Geliebter, A., Volkow, N. D., et al. (2011). Enhanced striatal dopamine release during food stimulation in binge eating disorder. *Obesity, 19*(8), 1601–1608.

Wang, S. B., Gray, E. K., Coniglio, K. A., et al. (2021). Cognitive rigidity and heightened attention to detail occur transdiagnostically in adolescents with eating disorders. *Eating Disorders, 29*(4), 408–420.

Wang, S. B., Jones, P. J., Dreier, M., Elliott, H., & Grilo, C. M. (2019). Core psychopathology of treatment-seeking patients with binge-eating disorder: A network analysis investigation. *Psychological Medicine, 49*(11), 1923–1928.

Waters, T. L., & Barrett, P. M. (2000). The role of the family in childhood obsessive-compulsive disorder. *Clinical Child and Family Psychology Review, 3*(3), 173–184. https://doi.org/10.1023/a:1009551325629.

Waters, A., Hill, A., & Waller, G. (2001). Bulimics' responses to food cravings: Is binge-eating a product of hunger or emotional state? *Behaviour Research and Therapy, 39*(8), 877–886.

Watson, H. J., & Bulik, C. M. (2013). Update on the treatment of anorexia nervosa: Review of clinical trials, practice guidelines and emerging interventions. *Psychological Medicine, 43*(12), 2477–2500. https://doi.org/10.1017/S0033291712002620.

Weltzin, T. E., Hsu, L. G., Pollice, C., & Kaye, W. H. (1991). Feeding patterns in bulimia nervosa. *Biological Psychiatry, 30*(11), 1093–1110.

Wentz, E., Gillberg, I. C., Anckarsäter, H., Gillberg, C., & Råstam, M. (2009). Adolescent-onset anorexia nervosa: 18-year outcome. *The British Journal of Psychiatry: The Journal of Mental Science, 194*(2), 168–174. https://doi.org/10.1192/bjp.bp.107.048686.

Wentz, E., Gillberg, C., Gillberg, I. C., & Råstam, M. (2001). Ten-year follow-up of adolescent-onset anorexia nervosa: Psychiatric disorders and overall functioning scales. *Journal of Child Psychology and*

Psychiatry and Allied Disciplines, 42(5), 613–622.

West, C. E., Goldschmidt, A. B., Mason, S. M., & Neumark-Sztainer, D. (2019). Differences in risk factors for binge eating by socioeconomic status in a community-based sample of adolescents: Findings from Project EAT. *International Journal of Eating Disorders, 52*(6), 659–668. https://doi.org/10.1002/eat.23079.

Wheaton, M. G., Galfalvy, H., Steinman, S. A., et al. (2016). Patient adherence and treatment outcome with exposure and response prevention for OCD: Which components of adherence matter and who becomes well? *Behaviour Research and Therapy, 85*, 6–12.

White, M. (1986). Negative explanation, restraint, and double description: A template for family therapy. *Family Process, 25*(2), 169–184.

Whitehead, M. R., & Suveg, C. (2016). Difficulties in emotion regulation differentiate depressive and obsessive-compulsive symptoms and their co-occurrence. *Anxiety, Stress, & Coping, 29* (5), 507–518.

Wilfley, D. E., Agras, W. S., Telch, C. F., et al. (1993). Group cognitive-behavioral therapy and group interpersonal psychotherapy for the nonpurging bulimic individual: A controlled comparison. *Journal of Consulting and Clinical Psychology, 61*(2), 296–305. https://doi.org/10.1037//0022-006x.61.2.296.

Wilfley, D. E., Welch, R. R., Stein, R. I., et al. (2002). A randomized comparison of group cognitive-behavioral therapy and group interpersonal psychotherapy for the treatment of overweight individuals with binge-eating disorder. *Archives of General Psychiatry, 59*(8), 713–721. https://doi.org/10.1001/archpsyc.59.8.713.

Wilfley, D. E., Welch, R. R., Stein, R. I., et al. (2013). A randomized controlled comparison of groupcognitive-behavioral therapy and group interpersonal therapy for the treatment ofoverweight individuals with binge-eating disorder. *Archives of General Psychiatry, 70*(9), 1061–1071.

Williams, M. T., Farris, S. G., Turkheimer, E., et al. (2011). Myth of the pure obsessional type in obsessive-compulsive disorder. *Depression and Anxiety, 28*(6), 495–500.

Williams, M. T., Mugno, B., Franklin, M., & Faber, S. (2013). Symptom dimensions in obsessive-compulsive disorder: Phenomenology and treatment outcomes with exposure and ritual prevention. *Psychopathology, 46*(6), 365–376.

Wilsdon, A., & Wade, T. D. (2006). Executive functioning in anorexia nervosa: Exploration of the role of obsessionality, depression and starvation. *Journal of Psychiatric Research, 40* (8), 746–754.

Wilson, G. T., Eldredge, K. L., Smith, D., & Niles, B. (1991). Cognitive-behavioral treatment with and without response prevention for bulimia. *Behaviour Research and Therapy, 29*(6), 575–583.

Wilson, G. T., Fairburn, C. C., Agras, W. S., Walsh, B. T., & Kraemer, H. (2002). Cognitive-behavioral therapy for bulimia nervosa: Time course and mechanisms of change. *Journal of Consulting and Clinical Psychology, 70*(2), 267–274. https://doi.org/10.1037/0022-006X.70.2.267.

Wilson, G. T., Grilo, C. M., & Vitousek, K. M. (2007). Psychological treatment of eating disorders. *American Psychologist, 62*(3), 199–216. https://doi.org/10.1037/0003-066X.62.3.199.

Wilson, G. T., Rossiter, E., Kleifield, E. I., & Lindholm, L. (1986). Cognitive-behavioral treatment of bulimia nervosa: A controlled evaluation. *Behaviour Research and Therapy, 24*(3), 277–288.

Wilson, G. T., Wilfley, D. E., Agras, W. S., & Bryson, S. W. (2010). Psychological treatments of binge eating disorder. *Archives of General Psychiatry, 67*(1), 94–101. https://doi.org/10.1001/archgenpsychiatry.2009.170.

Wilson, G. T., & Zandberg, L. J. (2012). Cognitive-behavioral guided self-help for eating disorders: Effectiveness and scalability. *Clinical Psychology Review, 32* (4), 343–357. https://doi.org/10.1016/j.cpr.2012.03.001.

Wilsdon, A., & Wade, T. D. (2006). Executive functioning in anorexia nervosa: Exploration of the role of obsessionality, depression and starvation. *Journal of Psychiatric Research, 40* (8), 746–754.

Wonderlich, S. A., Crosby, R. D., Engel, S. G., et al. (2017). Evidence-based treatment practices for eating disorders: Results from a national survey of clinicians. *International Journal of Eating Disorders, 50*(7), 743–752.

Wonderlich, S. A., Lilenfeld, L. R., Riso, L. P., Engel, S., & Mitchell, J. E. (2005). Personality and anorexia nervosa. *International journal of Eating Disorders, 37 Suppl*, S68–S89. https://doi.org/10.1002/eat.20120.

Woods, S. C., & Ramsay, D. S. (2011). Food intake, metabolism and homeostasis. *Physiology & Behavior, 104*(1), 4–7.

Wu, K. D., & Cortesi, G. T. (2009). Relations between perfectionism and obsessive-compulsive symptoms: Examination of specificity among the dimensions. *Journal of Anxiety Disorders, 23* (3), 393–400.

Yao, S., Kuja-Halkola, R., Thornton, L. M., et al. (2016). Familial liability for eating disorders and suicide attempts: Evidence from a population registry in Sweden. *JAMA Psychiatry, 73*(3), 284–291. https://doi.org/10.1001/jamapsychiatry.2015.2737.

Yilmaz, Z., Halvorsen, M., Bryois, J., et al. (2020). Examination of the shared genetic basis of anorexia nervosa and obsessive-compulsive disorder. *Molecular Psychiatry, 25*(9), 2036–2046. https://doi.org/10.1038/s41380-018-0115-4.

Zandian, M., Ioakimidis, I., Bergh, C., & Södersten, P. (2007). Cause and treatment of anorexia nervosa. *Physiology & Behavior, 92* (1–2), 283–290.

Zeeck, A., Herpertz-Dahlmann, B., Friederich, H. C., et al. (2018). Psychotherapeutic treatment for anorexia nervosa: A systematic review and network meta-analysis. *Frontiers in Psychiatry, 9*, 158. https://doi.org/10.3389/fpsyt.2018.00158.

Zeeck, A., Weber, S., Sandholz, A., et al. (2009). Inpatient versus day clinic treatment for bulimia nervosa: A randomized trial. *Psychotherapy and Psychosomatics, 78*(3), 152–160. https://doi.org/10.1159/000206869.

Zucker, N. L., LaVia, M. C., Craske, M. G., et al. (2019). Feeling and body investigators (FBI): ARFID division – An acceptance-based interoceptive exposure treatment for children with ARFID. *International Journal of Eating Disorders, 52*(4), 466–472.

Zvolensky, M. J., Vujanovic, A. A., Bernstein, A., & Leyro, T. (2010). Distress tolerance: Theory, measurement, and relations to psychopathology. *Current Directions in Psychological Science, 19*(6), 406–410.

Index